Managing Weight and Health

For Men and Women, Young and Old

Oskar Callin

Contents

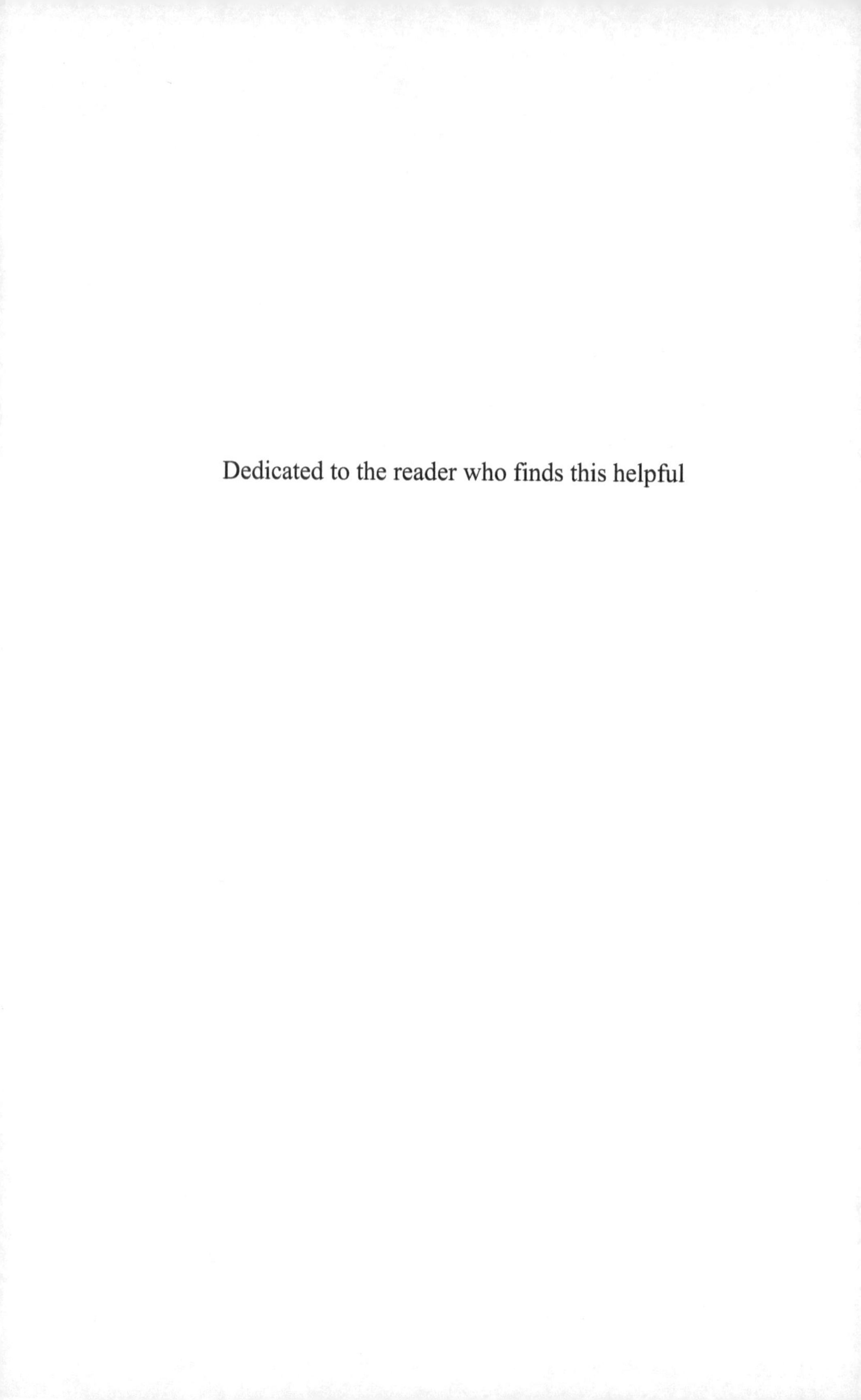

Dedicated to the reader who finds this helpful

Acknowledgements

WITHOUT Ivan Butler, this book would have been impossible to complete. He accepted the roughest of drafts without frown. An absolute professional.

I owe a lot to my friends and family too. If you have one true friend, you can consider yourself rich. I feel extremely fortunate because several people showed up for me when things were bad, without me even asking for it. I will always love you.

And finally, I also want to thank the people whose actions contributed to the hardest times of my life. I will always have love for you too. Even though I experienced suffering, I knew that the actions came from a place of love. And, thanks to those experiences, I was able to meet the love of my life. I believe that everything had to happen the way it did to lead me to you, Aremi. I love you.

Preface

My ambition with this book is to help people to take control of their weight and health. I'm repeatedly asked for advice about these matters because I have a lot of experience. My problem is that I can't explain everything that people need to know in a brief conversation. It breaks my heart to see people struggle with self-esteem because they don't know how to manage their physical bodies. Anyone can do it, but the right information can be hard to come by.

People *want* to be able to control their bodies, enough so that many share the experience of having starved themselves for months, or having initiated an extreme exercise routine, only to finally give up, ending up disheartened and heavier than before. People deserve to know how simple and enjoyable it can be to take control of their bodies. That's why I wanted to create this book. It's an extension of me in the sense that I can explain what *I know* and how I managed to get to where *I wanted to be*, which *you* can use in order to get to where *you want to be*.

I hope that 'my voice' comes through in this book. There's a multitude of ways to get to where one wants, but not every strategy will work for every person. My ambition is simply to share what *I know* in a format that's easily understandable and distributable. I've chosen to focus on the simplest, most universal strategies and methods that I've practiced myself for about a decade and a half. My belief is that that an understanding of a few fundamental aspects regarding weight and health will give any person the ability to control their own body's appearance and health.

This book is divided into three parts, although they're all related in some way. The first part is where I attempt to share many fundamentals regarding my perspective on weight, hunger, health, and fitness. The point of the first part is to illuminate how simple it really is to manage one's weight and health, and how essential it is to maintain a positive mindset.

The second part outlines the actual process of 'doing' what you need to do to transform. The way I see it, transforming/managing your weight and managing your health is a skill, just like playing a musical instrument or driving a car. My ambition is to teach you the skill of transforming so that you can use it any way you want. Just like with other skills, you need to practice them in real life.

The third part is about longevity. You'll learn throughout the book that you're on a journey, and that this journey is both tremendously exciting and enjoyable. It's therefore essential that we speak about how to keep on pursuing worthwhile goals without having to sacrifice the aspect of 'living life.' Managing weight and health isn't about always starving.

A lot of concepts and ideas will be repeated and revisited throughout this book. It's in part a by-product of the creative process of writing this book, but also, and more so, something I believe is a necessity. Understanding and learning is an individual process, and some examples might seem very concrete to one person while they completely go over someone else's head. With repetition and more repetition, my hope is that the ideas and mantras contained within this books start to infest the mind of the reader. I've come to think that voices inside of the head can be a good thing, at least as long as they are encouraging, positive, and truthful.

Although you'll be given my perspective on managing weight and health, you can rest assured that much of it is also based on the borrowed ideas from much smarter, more experienced people than myself. So essentially, this is just a collection of thoughts and ideas that I wish everyone knew, because people deserve to be healthy and feel beautiful.

Part 1

THE FUNDAMENTALS

Anyone Can Do It

It's my firm belief that *anyone* can be in control of how they look, feel and perform. It doesn't matter too much to me if this statement comes off as unrealistic or naive. As long as we're human, certain principles of (positive) body and health manipulation will apply to us all. You can be as much of a doubter as you please but practice the principles in this book and you'll see for yourself.

The reason for my stubborn belief isn't based on the fact that I learned to control my own performance and appearance. Rather, my conviction is rooted in me witnessing first-hand how replicable results are. The principles taught in this book are universal and transferrable. It doesn't matter if you're a twenty-something-year-old female wanting to compete in your first bikini competition, a thirty-something-year-old male who hasn't worked out in a decade, having worked up a gut you think is too big, or if you're a fifty-something-year-old divorcee who's given up all hope that you'll lose the excess 25-plus kg. (55-plus lb.) that's making your health and social life suffer.

The anonymous individuals just mentioned are some of the people that have come to me for advice. I'm not really the type of person who likes to give advice but offering my opinion and guidance has more and more started to feel like a duty. I would like to try to explain why.

One of the worst things I've witnessed started at a social gathering a few years back. It was summer time, and a neighborhood get-together was in session. People from all ages were present—kids, grown-ups, acquaintances, unknown but familiar faces, and friends.

All of a sudden, I overheard two couples catching up with each other. An acquaintance's dad and his partner were standing opposite an unknown couple that I assumed were old friends or neighbors. Right next to my acquaintance's dad was a middle-aged woman, his partner, having made an obvious effort to dress up for the occasion. The clothing, make-up and accessories were on point, and you could tell that this woman was having a good time. What I then happened to witness was how she received a compliment from the other woman in the company:

"You look fabulous. I really love your outfit!"

Before the compliment could be accepted, my acquaintance's dad replied for her with a chuckle:

"Thank you, but you should've seen her before she got pregnant," gesturing with his hands to form a thin line, right in front of his partner. Although my acquaintance's partner tried hard to attempt a smile, the cut was as irreversible as it was visible from afar.

Several evenings during a two-week period following this incident, I saw that same woman jogging around the lap where I usually took my walks. She would wear a pair of those neon-colored running shoes, which looked brand-new. She had a determined look on her face. Then, she just disappeared.

Years later, I still live in the same neighborhood, and I still see the woman from time to time. She wasn't even close to unhealthy-looking when the scene played out. It's obvious that her figure is a bit bigger now, however. What's worse is that her posture and radiance has completely changed. I still see her beside the same man at times, when they are sluggishly walking to- or from the local bar. She barely seems to say anything anymore. She mostly just looks at the ground, slouched. Defeated.

She's someone's mother, and she could just as well have been my own. I know what my parents have sacrificed for me and my brother, and they'll always be beautiful to us. No one could ever tell us that they're not good enough, and no person should ever be made to feel like they're not. That's part of why, since the episode played out, I've felt responsible to share what I know with the people who want advice about body transformation.

Arguing that the beer-bellied, semi-drunk of a man should be the one making an effort as he seems to care so much is logical, although I'm doubtful whether it will make much of a difference. This all-too-common dynamic is a real social problem, which I unfortunately don't know how to tackle.

What I *do* know, however, is how to help individuals from all walks of life to take control of their bodies. If that's an ambition of yours, rest assured it's doable. In this book I want to share how anyone can take control of their health and appearance without having to become an Instagram personality or full-time health freak.

I don't want to share what I know so that people can get validation from assholes like the one just described, or from anyone else. No, the reason is that I've seen what a sense of control does for people's confidence, and I've experienced it for myself too. Learning how to control the way you look and feel gives you a sense of confidence, independence and self-worth. You can validate yourself and say fuck off to everyone else, especially people that don't treat you with the respect you deserve.

Anyone *can* do this. I've witnessed it first-hand, and you'll see it for yourself if you try your best to follow the principles in this book. The book contains what I think everyone deserves to know about their bodies. I do feel like it's my duty to share it. Hopefully it's possible to understand why.

Being Conscious and Aware

This book will treat a multitude of ideas and concepts. Eventually, you'll know them all by heart, but you shouldn't worry about grasping everything right away. The first part of the book is as much an introduction to the fundamental concepts as it is a companion to revisit continually during weeks and years to come. Don't strive to implement anything until we get to the second part of the book. That's when you'll begin to act and start doing things with your diet.

Until we get there, please just try to read and absorb the ideas. Try to mentally prepare to act once we reach the next part. Once there, you'll have concrete instructions to follow. As long as you're prepared to adhere to the second part of the book, you'll achieve your results. Until then, read (and perhaps re-read) about the fundamentals contained within Part 1 until you feel ready to move on to the next part.

To start the book off, I would like to introduce you to a thought-provoking comparison that illuminates a fundamental assumption that influences the entire book: *we all just need to be more mindful about our food behavior.* Now, bear with me as I try to illustrate what uncritical food behavior looks like, and why we sometimes just need to stop for a second and think.

It doesn't take long to realize that Jay Cutler knows what he's doing when it comes to shaping his body:

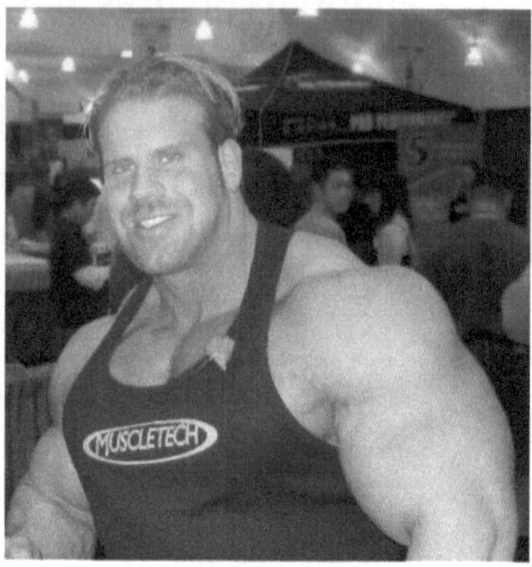

For anyone who hasn't been a world champion bodybuilder yet, it's only possible to intellectually understand what Mr. Cutler has done to achieve his results. Reaching the level Jay reached meant a twelve-year journey consisting of exercise four times a day, seven meals of measured and purposeful food, and regular naps. Sacrificing energy for recreation and socializing, or missing a single meal was completely unacceptable, so Jay invested close to all his twenty-four hours every day for twelve years to achieving what he did.

Grasping this investment intellectually is one thing, but could you imagine living the described lifestyle for twelve straight years, twenty-plus hours a day, pursuing world titles? Bodybuilders are interesting … the dedication they require is extreme.

Now, why do I bring up Jay Cutler? The idea is to highlight something quite astounding. Jay Cutler had to eat seven meals a day to feed his 260 to 290 lb. (118 to 132 kg.), depending on the season. It sounds extreme, and even most professional bodybuilders, in fact, don't get their frequency up to seven meals per day on such a consistent basis (that's why they're not world champions). However, Mark Bell, a particularly good influencer whom I highly recommend people to follow (he's everywhere on YouTube and other platforms), did some informal research, and he found something very thought-provoking: on average, Americans consume calories fifteen times a day.

Isn't that something? Just to clarify the potential confusion: eating a meal is of course equal to consuming calories, but so is having a cappuccino, for example, on your way to a meeting. A Starbucks cappuccino ranges from 80 to 150 calories, depending on size. Had you also eaten a Snickers bar before the exemplified meeting, that's an additional 250 calories to be added. Imagine consuming ten to twelve such and similar levels of calories throughout the day, and then having three to five normal meals. It's more extreme than Jay Cutler's meal frequency!

That John and Jane Doe struggle with weight and appearance is dependent on more than one factor. But the fact that they habitually consume calories twice as many times as a world champion bodybuilder is certainly one of them. My personal (albeit unscientific) speculation is this: John and Jane aren't aware of their habits. I only base this thought on anecdotal evidence, on the fact that I've been in the same situation myself, and that 99 percent of the people that have thus far come to me for guidance are just as unaware. I think awareness is one of the most important keys to gaining control over your body and its destiny (if not the most important). It's the first part of this book.

With mindfulness and awareness about the food we eat—about its calorie content and how these calories generally affect us—and a little bit of exercise, we (that is, you, me, John, and Jane) don't need much more to achieve our ideal bodies. Awareness, exercise, and consistency; those principles alone can get you as far as you want to go.

Formulas vs. Mindfulness

This book will show you how to be mindful about food rather than providing you with 'practical formulas' for 'optimal' fat loss or anything of that sort. What you should eat, and how much, depends on your personal goals and preferences. And, unless you've regularly met with a fitness professional for about a year, and that professional understands your body and goals just as well as you do (which is *extremely* rare), your best shot at making real, sustainable progress is to get in tune with your own body and learn the skill of transforming for yourself.

Your primary aim is to take the reins and accept complete responsibility for your transformation. You need to own the entire process. If this makes you feel afraid or left out, don't worry. I and many, many others have felt it too. Eventually, however, calm and confidence sets in. This is because results build confidence and certainty. If you consistently keep going after your calorie goals, which is something essential that you'll be learning about and will practice throughout this book, you *will* achieve results and progress. Doubting yourself for moments in time is completely normal, so don't worry about it.

To show what I mean, I refer you to Brené Brown's book, *Rising Strong: How the Ability to Reset Transforms the Way We Live, Love, Parent, and Lead*. Brown is a world-renowned social scientist, who speaks about overcoming adversity and big setbacks with The Rising Strong Process. In summary, the process is divided into three separate steps, each being mandatory. In the book, Brown shows how effective the process is, but she also explains how demanding the entire process can be to follow through. A very typical human tendency, which seems to hinder effective overcoming of adversity, is that most people skip the middle step, which perhaps is *the* most crucial step. The integral second step of The Rising Strong Process is where you take complete responsibility and ownership of your struggle and circumstances. Before owning the struggle, most people tend to want to solve their situation with the most comfortable means they can think of. Only when reaching a stage of acceptance of the fact that there's no easy fix, does the true way forward present itself.

The tendency to look for the easiest and most comfortable way to resolution of a situation is a very human trait. In relation to the body transformation journey, the 'easy, comfortable way' usually equates to magical diet pills, fat-burning green teas, or crash diets. The true way forward, however, is the mindful and responsible path. We need to understand and account for what we eat and stay with the plan until we change goals. The new goal is then what decides what and how much to eat, and new targets are pursued until ...

Owning responsibility for the transformation, and accepting the path, is the true way forward. The more you get to know yourself, the better you can control your progress. No external product will guarantee your progress—you and your mind are the magic ingredients. You'll be very proud once you manage to get to the place where you own and control your body. It's independence of the highest order and, unfortunately, it's something that appears very difficult and rare to achieve in today's society. That's nonetheless the direction in which we're heading—towards control, ownership and independence.

Keeping it Simple

After roughly sixteen years of gathering personal and anecdotal experience relating to conscious eating and exercise, I would say that the most common reason people fail to achieve results in the body transformation department is because the process appears complex. This is also what used to stop me from achieving results. I couldn't decide which of the diets/tactics/fads/magical pills seemed best, so I tried and failed them all (a process that took a bit longer than two years). So, I'll tell you about the crucial shift in mindset that turned my failing self into an achieving self instead, which is something you'll also be able to do.

The initial usage of the phrase 'appears complex' above was intentional. The process of achieving transformative results really isn't complicated. There's an issue, however, in that the simple solution is hidden in a swamp of complexity. In order for us to achieve results, we need to find our way out of the metaphorical swamp. To do this, we need to talk about the current issue of complexity from the ground up, and then talk about the solution that leads to results.

The Issue

A paradigm is a thought pattern that guides our worldview. See the illustrative picture here:

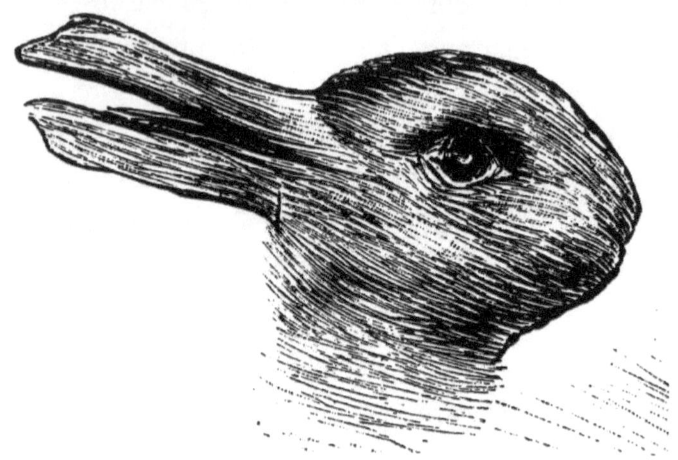

Is this a duck or a bunny? It can be both. It's what we choose to see that matters. The same goes for many other areas in life. Our paradigm—our worldview—shapes what we see and experience, and very often this paradigm has been created without our own conscious influence.

What are the odds that we automatically have the soundest understanding about health and fitness? Is it not reasonable to speculate that movies, magazines, and various luminaries have affected our understanding of what it takes to achieve a healthy and appealing body? Is it possible that a bombardment of messages saying either that a transformation is 'easy, just take this pill' or that it's 'impossible, unless you do this complicated diet' have confused us? I think so.

What do most people think it takes to achieve their ideal body? What paradigm guides their reasoning? Most people think that an ideal body is the result of controlled starvation, immense activity, odd weight loss strategies, etc. I think this is the reason people *see* the process of achieving the ideal body as complicated (pun intended).

In reality, you can rest assured that it isn't, but when you constantly hear different voices treating a multitude of topics of varying relevance—that is, anything from odd trends to body recomposition, to targeted fat reduction (which doesn't actually work), to super diets, to cutting and bulking, to name just a few—it's difficult to grasp what information is applicable and important to you and your goals. Confusion is a given. I believe this is one of the main reasons people fail to achieve results and transform their bodies.

There's an overflow of information, much of it unnecessarily complex or even irrelevant. The current paradigm portrays 'complexity' as the true condition of health and fitness, and it's misleading. The best solution to this problem, at least from what I've found through my years of experience, is to introduce a new paradigm that replaces complexity with simplicity.

The Solution

How cliché it is to say that mindset is a fundamental key, but it's nonetheless true. That's why I want you to forget all of the complex methods, trends, and buzzwords mentioned above, as well as all of the future ones. In fact, forget everything you may already know about creating an ideal body! The old paradigm—the paradigm that influences you to think that a body transformation is a complex matter—we're now going to shift.

From now on, you're to understand that a transformation is the *simplest thing in the world*. How simple? It's as simple as mastering the art of *calorie counting* and striving for *one goal at a time*. So, the only two thoughts you should let occupy your mind from now on are these:

1. Your key to your ideal body lies in your ability to count and track *calories*.

2. Your only goal currently is to *lose weight*, nothing else.

The significance of the above can't be overstated. These mental guidelines should infest your mind until you unquestionably act in accordance with them. Their pursuit will become your new religion, your new paradigm. I'll cover the first part, the one having to do with calorie counting, later, so don't worry about it just yet. Right now, you need to understand why your only objective is to *lose weight*.

Before we go into *how* you lose weight, we need to understand *why* we focus on this aspect. As I mentioned previously, we need to talk about the correct subject matter in the right order. What do I mean when I say that? Well, if we for instance were to build a house from scratch, it would be best to focus on the blueprint and how to mix the concrete for the foundation, rather than what brand of charcoal grill to place on the lawn. Although a nice grill has an important and rightful place in a house, it isn't a relevant topic to talk about at this point in time. With a solid foundation, we can build a house, and then we can start furnishing and decorating it.

As this relates to your body transformation, weight loss is the most relevant concept to talk about right now. When we talk about losing weight, please understand that we're also connoting the by-products of losing weight as well—that is, the fat loss, improved appearance, and other general health benefits that come from having a healthier body weight—however, the wording we're to use is 'weight loss' and nothing else. It's our foundation and succeeding in this area leads to the other benefits just mentioned, automatically.

So, weight loss is what we strive for, and it's the indicator of our results. If the weight goes down over time, we're winning. If weight is going up, we're doing it wrong, and need to course correct. It's as simple as that.

Once we do get our weight going in the right direction, things will start happening to our body's fat distribution and appearance. This is the part where the change isn't only appearing on the scale, but also becomes visible in the mirror. To understand what you'll see in the mirror once you make progress, and what you can expect yourself to look like over time, we need to talk a bit more in depth about fat in the following pages.

Basics About Body Fat

Some knowledge about body fat is necessary for you to create reasonable expectations. How much body fat you currently have, and how little body fat you need to look great, is important information you need to understand. I'm not trying to say you need exact, pinpoint precision, but you do need to understand enough about body fat so that your guestimations are in the ballpark, however.

Here are a few rules of thumb:

- Most people think they're a lower body fat than they actually are.

- Most people look great at 12 percent body fat.

- If you carry more than an average amount of muscle, 15 percent body fat is low enough to look great.

For women, the numbers are skewed upward by around 5 percent. With the above rules of thumb in mind, take a look at the following picture portraying Rich Froning Jr., who has won the title of 'Fittest Man on Earth' four times. When competing, Froning is likely around 12 percent body fat. If you weren't primed with the previous information, what body fat percentage do you think you would have guessed?

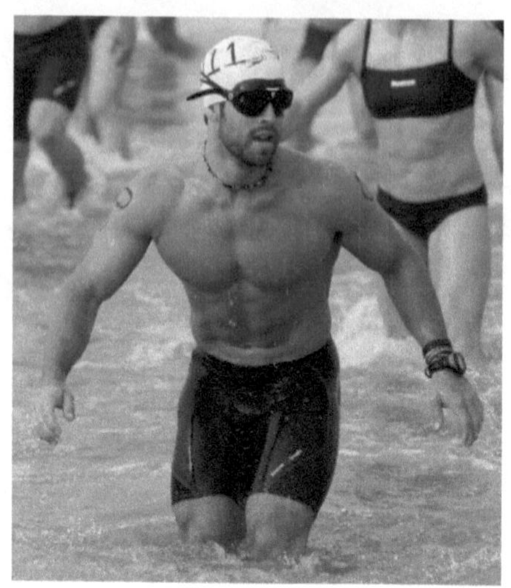

Now take a look at the next picture. It's a side-by-side comparison of Swedish bodybuilder Robert Berg.

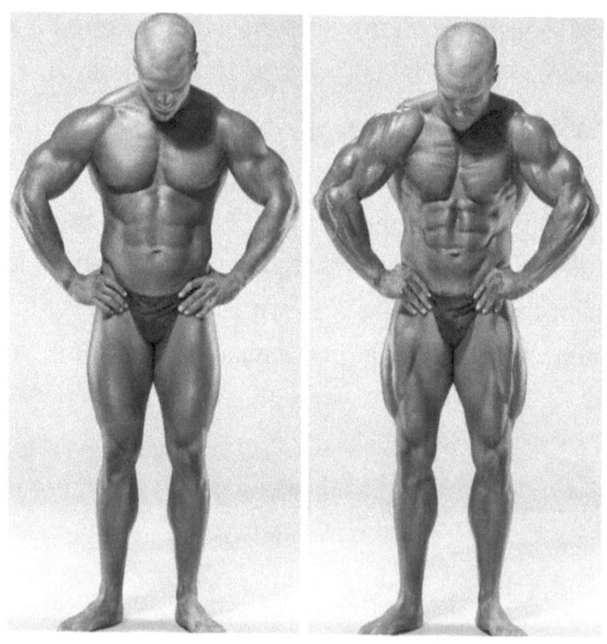

The two pictures were taken within about one second of each other. First, the difference looks drastic. Second, the body fat percentage is around 8 percent. What body fat percentage would you have guessed if you only saw one of the pictures?

The internet is great but using it to find accurate body fat estimations can be trickier than it should be. As you can probably tell just from looking at the exemplified pictures, different lighting, angles, and also photo filters can make a *huge* difference to how a person looks in a photo. That's why the rules of thumb are useful. They're intended to guide you and calibrate your expectations. I hope the exemplified images help convey the somewhat weird relation between body fat and appearance.

What I want you to take away from these examples is that the mirror and your personal opinion is what ultimately should matter to you. Your body fat percentage can be 'this' or 'that' but what do you actually want to look like?

An ideal look is a subjective matter, and you can't be wrong when choosing yours. What's essential, however, is that you manage your expectations when it comes to what you need to do to get there, and what a reasonable timeframe looks like.

Most people that show me a photo of a person they think has an ideal body ask, "Do you think I can achieve this? Is it too far off for me?" But they can reach far beyond the ideal they have in mind. Even though this is the case, most people never get to see their ideal bodies in the flesh. The reason, nine times out of ten, is because an understanding of the requisite timeframe is uncalibrated or lacking. This is why it's absolutely essential that we deeply understand everything about the word 'patience' within the context of this book.

Patience

Say that you, for instance, learn the following: I can consume x calories without gaining weight. If x calories keeps you at the same weight, you understand that x-200 calories should decrease your body weight over time. You thus decide on the following action: for the next two weeks, I'll consume x-200 calories.

The math is ridiculously simple. In fact, it's so simple it feels like a joke. Trust me, though, it isn't. Why such a simple concept tends to be misunderstood and misused is due to over-excitement. Although it might not appear so at first sight, a 200-calorie reduction is a significant reduction. You very rarely (basically never if you're not an athlete with performance-related or appearance-related goals) need a larger adjustment than this. In fact, my personal opinion is that you should very rarely (basically almost never) decrease or increase your calories by more than 400 at a time, and I also think that you should be ready to stay with your chosen calorie adjustment for at least two weeks before you consider your next calorie target.

With these guidelines in mind, you would only change your calorie target once every other week or so, depending on whether you're making progress in the weight loss department or not. And keep in mind that weight loss isn't a static function. You want to achieve a *trend* of weight loss. A two-week period of consistently meeting your calorie goal will show you whether the trend is going in the right direction or not. Adjusting your calories should be based on the trend, and the changes should be of 200-ish magnitudes.

This brings us to a vital point. You can't speed up the transformation progress by drastically reducing your calories. I want you to understand that losing weight is much like giving birth to a baby. Regardless of what you do, it will take nine months until the baby arrives. You can be as intimate as you want for as many times as you wish during these nine months, but it will *not* change how much time the process takes. By the same reasoning, enormous calorie deficits won't benefit your body transformation, neither will excessive activity.

Trying to shortcut the system does more harm than good. Your appearance *will* change over time, and you need to have patience. Nine times out of ten, a transformation takes two to six months if done correctly (that is, steadily and patiently). A few months is nothing in relation to the span of a normal life. We'll go on an actual transformation journey in Part 2 of this book, so prepare mentally to give yourself a few months to learn the skill of transformation. If you learn this skill, you'll always be able to look the way you want.

You truly need to let the process take its time, though. To further drive home this point, I would like to speak briefly about the reasons why activity won't equal additional results. If that were the case, lots of people with a good work ethic would be in the shape of their lives. To illustrate my point, please have a look at the following picture, which shows that it's very plain to see that you *can't* outrun an uncritical food behavior.

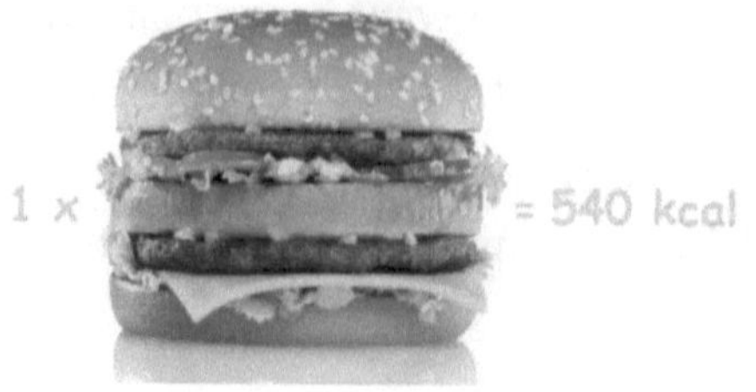

Being unaware of how many calories one consumes, and not knowing how much time would have to be spent to undo the calories, leads to excess weight. This is why you just need to start making conscious choices. A Big Mac can fit anyone's diet, so that's not the issue. The issue is that most people are unaware of what they eat, and how much *time* (not *activity*) a transformation takes.

Perfect, Optimal, Enough

We won't be discussing much about perfection or optimal procedures in this book. This is for a few reasons. To start with, the former ideal doesn't really exist. A perfect day may be achieved, but perfect weeks, months, and years? Not so much. Perfection is an ideal that often does more harm than good. We as humans are wired to give negative occurrences more meaning than positive ones; it's called negativity bias. If perfection is the ideal, then a small slip can induce a sense of failure, even though such a conclusion is fundamentally untrue. To strive for excellence is one thing, but perfection is something different. Any guiding framework other than 'perfection' is more suitable for our intents and purposes.

So, what about the second term 'optimal procedures' then? It's a better framework than perfection, but still quite irrelevant for our intents and purposes. Optimal procedures may be useful when fine-tuning the body for high-end endeavors, but they aren't needed even then. The last few weeks before getting ready to go on stage for a competition, or when breaking new ground and increasing strength as an advanced lifter, many people start looking for optimal procedures to use. However, 'doing enough consistently' will be more useful than 'being optimal for a while,' even at very high levels.

It's important that 'enough' is well understood because it looks like it means 'half-assed' when put next to terms like perfection and optimal. 'Enough' isn't a word for the complacent, regardless of the first impression it leaves. It simply means that you meet the criteria for your most important goals, every single day, consistently.

Depending on what you want to achieve and what level you're at, there are one to four goals that you need to handle on a consistent basis, which I cover in the following section, but the one thing that always needs to be in check, for everyone from beginners to professionals, is the food-related goal. Food and diet determine how our bodies react to exercise, as well as how it looks. Some people need to gain weight, some need to lose weight. The most important goal is the calories. Where the calories come from is up to you to decide, depending on how you want to feel mentally and physically, and what you want to achieve exercise-wise.

In relation to 'enough,' doing enough means that you consistently meet the calorie target you've set up. Even if some days are tough, you meet your target calories. That's what doing enough means. You do what you know you must do. Any other accomplishments during any given day are a bonus, and that's extra pride for you to enjoy. If you don't miss the targets you know you have to hit, you've done enough, and you deserve to go to bed fulfilled and satisfied with yourself.

Four Goals

When talking about doing enough, there's really only four things in total you would ever need to worry about achieving. Most often, it's even less than that. If you consistently do 'enough' in three out of the four areas we're about to discuss, you would be doing everything in your power to achieve your highest level of fitness, health, and appearance. This means that you would be on track to pursue the best physique your genetics allow for, and that you wouldn't leave anything of this pursuit to chance. Not everyone has this aspiration, however, and very often two out of the four goals are more than sufficient for most people.

Before detailing the three most important parts of the equation (the fourth isn't as important), I want to point out that I'm not trying to say that you should or need to implement everything immediately. Whatever you implement should be a lifelong endeavor, just as tracking and being mindful about food is going to become. Therefore, don't rush into anything. Results won't come any quicker; they still come from consistency. Make sure you've got goal number one down before you think about another goal.

With that said, goal number one is being in control of your food. There's no way around the fact that we need to be aware of what we eat. This awareness is what allows us to control what our bodies look like, and how they perform. If you know how to track your calories, weight, and judge how your appearance changes (via pictures or the mirror), then you're in control of your body's appearance. If you're also mindful about *where* your calories come from—candy or carrots, for instance—you have the means to control your performance and wellbeing. Food is number one, regardless of whether you're an athlete or a business professional.

Here's where it gets interesting. I have now exercised for around 16 years, so it's not unlikely that I'm favorably biased towards working out. Even so, I *still* put exercise as the number two goal, and it comes a close second to food. If it hadn't been for the fact that excess calories can outdo all the hard work that's put into exercise, I would have put exercise as number one. As we've just seen, however, that's not the case. We can't use exercise to outwork consuming too many calories. The excess calories won't transform into muscle or increased endurance, just fat.

However, exercise is still *the* health potion of health potions. There are too many beneficial effects from exercise to list here. The most common misconception is that exercise uses energy and leads to a deficiency of energy for other daily tasks, but that isn't right. Regular exercise leads to *more* energy. That's the only way to put it; it's simply in your best interest to implement exercise in your life, sooner rather than later.

Doing the same exercise for fifteen to twenty minutes a day is plenty to start with. Such a routine could even last you a lifetime. If you increase the intensity and length of the individual sessions, you could get away with four sessions a week doing heavier basic exercises, such as the bench press and squat. As I said, this is in your best interest.

However, and this is a big 'however,' don't start exercising until you're ready to be consistent with it. Make sure you have the first goal, food/calories, down to a routine before starting to implement the habit of exercise. If you just get number one and two down as lifelong habits, you can reach at least 80 percent of your potential, and that would be immensely successful.

The third goal is cardio, which serves two purposes. The primary purpose is that cardio is extremely healthy. Your body and mind will simply perform and feel better with a healthy cardiovascular system. Losing a hundred pounds will certainly feel better than improving your cardio ever will, so food is number one, but when you're down to a normal weight, cardio will start increasing wellbeing, while wellbeing from loss of bodyweight diminishes.

The second purpose, or perhaps utility, of cardio is that it can help the process of losing body fat. During the last three to four weeks of a transformation, added cardio usually helps the transformation process along. So, cardio can supply better health and appearance, but remember, it's not the primary priority—food and exercise come first by a long shot. Long walks, jogging, high-intensity interval training (HIIT), and swimming are all examples of cardio. I prefer long walks (about forty minutes), but you should do the one you prefer.

Finally, the fourth goal, which some people like to include in their routine, is skincare and tanning. Some people like to use face masks, creams, and tanning to get a specific look. A skincare routine combined with peaking during a transformation process can be highly motivating. Usually, you look the best you ever have during this period. So, if you've got your food, exercise, and cardio down, and you're about to 'peak' (be the lowest amount of body fat, be your most muscular, etc.), you may want to consider taking extra good care of your skin during this period. Small things matter when the big things are done consistently.

In Case You Want to Exercise

I have many opinions on exercise, but they depend on context and what the purpose of the exercise is. However, I do have a few general guiding principles, which fit most everyone.

- I'm a firm believer in the fact that the best exercise is the one you do. Even a ten-minute workout is great stuff if it's happening consistently. My recommendation is that you search for something you can see yourself doing for a long time without burning out, because it helps consistency.

- I believe the activity of exercise should be super easy to enact, especially for beginners and intermediates (that is, those who have less than five years' experience of consistent exercise), although this can apply to others too. Push-ups, pull-ups, squats, dips, and long walks can all be performed in a few minutes at the house, and that's my favorite type of 'easy,' when there are no practical or time-related restrictions at all. The less complicated, the better. It's setting you up to win!

- Lastly, I believe in developing a solid foundation to start with. Not everyone will have the same ultimate goal, but I believe strength training is where to start. A patient endeavor (not risking any injuries) to increase strength won't only translate to heavier weights lifted or more repetitions made, progress that's simple to track and steer, but strength training generally leads to more muscle on men, firmer bodies for women, and stronger joints and bones for both. Strength isn't only correlated with a specific appearance, but also with mental and physical health. A strong and solid foundation is the primary aim of exercise, in my opinion. So, to summarize:

1. Consistent exercise is the bread and butter, the 80 percent piece of the cake.

2. If the exercise is very practical to enact, that's a huge relief, and you set yourself up to win.

3. Becoming stronger is the primary objective because it gives you a solid foundation that not only improves your physical and mental health for the long term, but also improves your appearance.

Before continuing, an important notion needs to be discussed. Many women express a fear that strength training will cause them to look bulky. That's just not the case, and women shouldn't worry about it. I understand that these words may need backing up, since I'm not a woman myself. Therefore, I would like to refer women to influencers such as Meg Gallagher (megsquats) and Holly Baxter. Both women utilize strength training, and it doesn't detract from their femininity.

The Bench Press

The bench press is a great strength-building exercise for both women and men. Although it may not seem logical at first, once mastered, the bench press stimulates the entire body at the same time. With practice, the legs, abs, lats, chest, and arms all become involved simultaneously. Comparatively speaking, this helps to lift heavier weights than exercises such as tricep extensions and shoulder laterals. That's why the bench press is one of the best and most effective exercises for strength there is.

It usually doesn't take much to convince a man to do the bench press, because it's a fun exercise that's known for building the upper body, which most men tend to prioritize. However, the bench press isn't only an exercise dedicated to appearance, but also, and perhaps more so, to strength and health improvements. That's why the bench press is universally beneficial for both men and women.

Now, I don't want to try to convince anyone to do anything they don't want to do, but I'll say this: it's really, really arduous to build muscle, even for men with loads more testosterone than women. One simply doesn't wake up 'too big' suddenly. There's time to course correct if things get out of hand, although it's doubtful they ever will. The fear of looking built, instead of toned, has steered many women away from the bench press. That fear is over-dimensioned. If you don't want to do the bench press, that's perfectly okay, but you may miss out on some impressive results if you don't ever try it.

Finally, I would like to give some realistic bench press goals to strive for. Men should aim to perform a 100 kg. (220 lb.) bench press repetition. Usually, such an endeavor takes one to three years to achieve. Women, within a similar timeframe, should aim for a 50 kg. (110 lb.) bench press repetition. The most important rule is that you don't get injured, so pay attention to your body and be patient. I recommend Mark Bell's YouTube channels ('Mark Bell — Super Training Gym' and 'Mark Bell's Power Project') as a source of useful information about the bench press and lifting in general.

The Squat

Funnily enough, the squat often divides men and women in the opposite way the bench press does. From my experience, women tend to prefer good lower body development to good upper body development, and squats are arguably the best exercise for building a solid lower body, both strength-wise and appearance-wise.

Squats happen to be one of the toughest exercises there is, which probably explains why many shy away from them. The range of motion is many times longer than the bench press, and the exercise itself takes a lot of practice before it stops feeling awkward and hurting, etc. The list goes on. All speed bumps aside, however, a well-executed squat is a super-good exercise, which, to an even greater extent than the bench press, stimulates the entire body at the same time. Mike O'Hearn (also known as 'Titan') said he used to count his squat workouts as 'abs' too.

Squats and deadlifts (explained below) are the exercises where you'll be able to handle the most amount of weight, which means that they'll build a lot of strength if pursued diligently. Again, Mark Bell's YouTube channels are the places I recommend you visit for guidance. All I want to say, or perhaps repeat, is that you must avoid getting injured. This can't be stressed enough. Other than that, here are a few goals to pursue during the coming one to three years:

- Men should strive to perform one 140 kg. (308 lb.) squat.
- Women should strive to perform one 80kg. (176 lb.) squat.

The Deadlift

The deadlift is the exercise during which most people will be able to lift the heaviest amounts of weight and, naturally, this means it's a tremendous strength builder. The exercise itself can be somewhat tricky to master, and I therefore suggest you approach it with caution. Staying away from injury is of even higher importance than progress in the strength department. Again, Mark Bell's YouTube channels are major sources of information and guidance.

The deadlift builds the entire body, and in combination with the bench press and the squat, your body's natural strengths and weaknesses will be revealed as you become increasingly exposed to this type of exercise. Some will notice they're stronger in their lower body than upper body. Some will notice they're good at shaping their arms, while others notice their shoulders responding well to the exercise. With the deadlift, squat, and bench, you've got most of what you need your entire exercising life.

As I said, approach the deadlift with caution. Then, continue with patience, just as you would the other exercises. These are some numbers to aim for during the coming three years of doing the deadlift:

- Men who practice the deadlift for a few years can usually pull around 160 kg. (352 lb.) for two or three repetitions, and that's a good target to aim for.

- Women who practice the deadlift can usually pull around 80 kg. (176 lb.) for two or three repetitions, and that's the target to keep in mind and strive for.

Bodyweight Exercises

The squat and the bench press are great exercises, and I highly recommend them. However, if you don't want to commit to a gym membership yet, or if you don't already have the equipment at home, there are some great alternatives that will serve you extremely well.

Bodyweight exercises are even more practical than the squat and the bench press, and practicing just a few of the best bodyweight exercises alone can take a beginner very close to advanced levels of strength, if not all the way there, but it depends more on genetics. Pull-ups, chin-ups, dips, push-ups, lunges, and wall sits are great exercises that you can perform anytime and almost anywhere. Here are some lifetime goals to strive for:

- Men should strive to be able to do three sets of ten repetitions of pull-ups or chin-ups. For dips and push-ups, three sets of twenty repetitions is the goal.

- Women should strive to be able to do three sets of five repetitions of pull-ups or chin-ups. For dips and push-ups, three sets of ten repetitions is the goal.

- Women and men should both strive to be able to do fifty walking lunges in a row, and a two-minute wall sit.

Bodyweight exercises are a good substitute for barbells and dumbbells, and they can serve you for a lifetime. Even doing just one of the mentioned exercises per day, which takes around five minutes, is great stuff. The best exercise is the one you do, and consistency is key.

At this point, most of the fundamentals have now been introduced and expounded upon. Although it's not yet time to get active, we're now about to get introduced to a few practical skills as well. You'll learn about using these in real life throughout Part 2, so this is still just theoretical. When you're in the practical part of the book, however, you can always go back to this part if you need assistance or guidance.

Necessary Skills

Did you know that an estimated 95 percent of our actions are automatic and unintentional? Often our eating, drinking, and socializing selves are just us operating on autopilot. If you're like me and most other people, you weren't lucky enough to be born with an autopilot that's conducive to an ideal appearance and super-healthy food habits. Just think about John and Jane Doe from the earlier chapter. Most of us have a similar setup, where we don't actively reflect about what we're eating. Although that's often unintentional and 'just happened,' it's tremendously common, and it's one of the major reasons most of us have extra weight we want to get rid of.

Fortunately, it's very possible to reconfigure the autopilot. In fact, with a little conscious initial effort on your behalf, your autopilot could consist of enjoyable *and* productive habits that automatically get you to where you want to be health-wise and appearance-wise. This is what we'll be pursuing in Part 2. For now, however, we'll only be introduced to the *idea* of rewiring the autopilot.

The first step that must be taken, which is absolutely essential, is this: *you need to become aware of how your current autopilot is set up*. Before even thinking about any body-altering solutions, you must understand *the nature* of your personal situation. If you're a person that struggles with hunger, we could, for instance, devise a strategy where foods of greater volume are prioritized, whereas if you struggle with time restraints and too often are forced to eat calorie-dense fast foods, we could instead go for a practical solution where portable eating is facilitated. 'Different strokes for different folks,' essentially.

The key is that *you* understand what *your* situation is. You need *awareness*.

How do you reach understanding and awareness? By tracking how much you eat per day—your calories. It's truly as simple as that. You will understand why as you get further into the book. At this point in time, however, you absolutely shouldn't worry about anything other than absorbing the ideas that are presented. Don't start counting calories yet, and don't start changing anything about your normal eating behavior. This is important. We'll get to this in Part 2.

Once you're out in the field, that's when the calorie counting starts for real. At that time, it's likely that you want to go back to this section of the book. So, for now, feel free to read about these skills superficially. You can go back here later on, as many times as you please.

Counting Calories

Before going into detail on how I want you to count calories, I need to point a few things out:

- **Forget**—I want you to get a fresh start. Hence, I want you to try your hardest to forget everything you've previously heard about calorie counting.

- **Don't be fooled**—Don't let anyone trick you into thinking calorie counting is difficult or time-consuming. It's simple. Worst case, you might need a week or two to get used to it, as already mentioned. But once you *do* get used to it, it's the simplest thing in the world.

- **No macronutrients**—I want you to especially ignore everything related to 'macros.' Although we'll touch upon this topic further on in the book, it will never be a primary concern for us. You'll gradually learn more and more about why common sense and calories will be what we focus on, not micronutrients.

The reason why the above preparatory conditions are mentioned is because it's tremendously important that you understand that we only want to learn how to count *calories*. It will become even more clear why we only care about calories in Part 2, but for now, just know that calorie counting is prioritized because it, alone, will bring you most of your results.

Think of the Pareto principle: 80 percent of your results will come from 20 percent of the effort/input. Calorie counting is one of those fundamental 20 percent principles. Get this single ability down, and you'll have 80 percent of what you need to achieve and keep your ideal body.

In the following pages you will encounter three calorie counting methods. Master these and you're set for life.

Method #1: Using Food Labels

Imagine you're on your way to the gym. Since you've been keeping up with fitness magazines and luminaries from the industry lately, you decide to consume one of the protein bars you saw recommended in an ad. Here's what the label looks like:

PROTEIN BAR 80g

Nutrition Facts	Amount/Serving	% DV**	Amount/Serving	% DV**
Serving Size: 1 bar (80g)	**Total Fat** 13g	**20%**	**Total Carbohydrate** 32g	**11%**
Servings Per Container: 1	Sat. Fat 7g	**35%**	Dietary Fiber 1g	**4%**
Calories 320	*Trans* Fat 0g		Sugars 5g	
Fat Cal. 110	**Cholesterol** 10mg	**3%**	Sugar Alcohol 19g	
	Sodium 160mg	**7%**	**Protein** 26g	
** Percent Daily Values (DV) are based on a 2,000 calorie diet.	Vitamin A 2% •	Vitamin C 0% •	Calcium 15% •	Iron 15%

INGREDIENTS: Protein Blend (Cross-Flow Microfiltered Whey Protein Isolate, Soy Protein Isolate, Whey Protein Concentrate, Milk Protein Isolate), High Protein Milk Chocolate Coating (Maltitol, Palm Kernel Oil, Whey Protein Concentrate, Sugar, Cocoa Powder, Soy Lecithin and Vanillin), Maltitol, High Protein Peanut Butter Coating (Maltitol, Palm Kernel Oil, Partially Defatted Peanut Flour, Milk Protein Isolate, Sodium Caseinate, Salt, Soy Lecithin and Natural Flavor), Glycerin, Granola (Whole Grain Rolled Oats, Whole Grain Rolled Wheat, Brown Sugar, Canola Oil, Coconut, Whey, Oat Flour, Almonds and Honey), Gelatin, Protein Crisps (Soy Protein Isolate, Tapioca Starch and Salt), Sweetened Condensed Skim Milk, Peanuts, Water, Peanut Butter (Peanuts, Salt), Peanut Flour, High Oleic Sunflower Oil, Butter, Soy Lecithin, Cornstarch, Vanilla Extract, Salt, Caramel Color. **ALLERGENS:** Contains Milk, Soy, Peanuts, Tree Nuts (Almonds and Coconut) and Wheat. This product is produced in a facility with Soy, Dairy, Egg and Wheat Ingredients, Peanuts, Seeds, Fish and Tree Nuts.

In my opinion, the label looks frighteningly informative. My spontaneous reaction is that this must be complicated. Take a minute to think about what you feel when you see the label. Complicated, right? Here's the thing, however: we're only looking for one key piece of information, nothing else. Here's what we're interested in:

PROTEIN BAR 80g

Nutrition Facts	Amount/Serving	% DV**	Amount/Serving	% DV**
Serving Size: 1 bar (80g)	**Total Fat** 13g	**20%**	**Total Carbohydrate** 32g	**11%**
Servings Per Container: 1	Sat. Fat 7g	**35%**	Dietary Fiber 1g	**4%**
Calories 320	*Trans* Fat 0g		Sugars 5g	
Fat Cal. 110	**Cholesterol** 10mg	**3%**	Sugar Alcohol 19g	
** Percent Daily Values (DV) are based on a 2,000 calorie diet.	**Sodium** 160mg	**7%**	**Protein** 26g	
	Vitamin A 2% • Vitamin C 0% • Calcium 15% • Iron 15%			

INGREDIENTS: Protein Blend (Cross-Flow Microfiltered Whey Protein Isolate, Soy Protein Isolate, Whey Protein Concentrate, Milk Protein Isolate), High Protein Milk Chocolate Coating (Maltitol, Palm Kernel Oil, Whey Protein Concentrate, Sugar, Cocoa Powder, Soy Lecithin and Vanillin), Maltitol, High Protein Peanut Butter Coating (Maltitol, Palm Kernel Oil, Partially Defatted Peanut Flour, Milk Protein Isolate, Sodium Caseinate, Salt, Soy Lecithin and Natural Flavor), Glycerin, Granola (Whole Grain Rolled Oats, Whole Grain Rolled Wheat, Brown Sugar, Canola Oil, Coconut, Whey, Oat Flour, Almonds and Honey), Gelatin, Protein Crisps (Soy Protein Isolate, Tapioca Starch and Salt), Sweetened Condensed Skim Milk, Peanuts, Water, Peanut Butter (Peanuts, Salt), Peanut Flour, High Oleic Sunflower Oil, Butter, Soy Lecithin, Cornstarch, Vanilla Extract, Salt, Caramel Color. **ALLERGENS:** Contains Milk, Soy, Peanuts, Tree Nuts (Almonds and Coconut) and Wheat. This product is produced in a facility with Soy, Dairy, Egg and Wheat Ingredients, Peanuts, Seeds, Fish and Tree Nuts.

Simple, right? One entire bar contains 320 calories. So, if you ate two bars, you would consume 640 calories. If you only ate half a bar, you would consume 160 calories. Simple math. This, and only this, is what I want you to learn how to track—the number of calories you consume. When using food labels and consuming 'full entities' (for example, one protein bar, two bags of peanuts, or three bags of pre-packaged baby carrots), this method is both incredibly simple and highly practical. You just add up the calories and get on with your life. It's that simple!

Method #2: Food Scale

The food scale is often used in combination with labels. Imagine you buy a bag of uncooked rice, for instance. You would likely not consume the entire 'entity' (the full bag) in one meal. Hence, you use the food scale to calculate the number of calories your meal will contain. So, imagine you want to eat a substantial portion of rice, and that this is what our exemplary food label looks like:

Nutrition Facts

Serving Size 100g

Amount Per Serving

Calories 370	Calories from Fat 24

	% Daily Value*
Total Fat 3g	4%
Saturated Fat 1g	3%
Cholesterol 0mg	0%
Sodium 7mg	0%
Total Carbohydrate 77g	26%
Dietary Fiber 4g	14%
Sugars 1g	
Protein 8g	

Vitamin A	0%	Vitamin C	0%
Calcium	2%	Iron	8%

*Percent Daily Values are based on a 2000 calorie diet. Your daily values may be higher or lower depending on your calorie needs.

Let's say you pour a generous pile of dry, uncooked rice into a bowl, and that the scale says 141 g. Knowing what you know about calorie counting and using the label above, the calorie count will be:

> *1.41 × 370 = 521.7 calories*

It really is as simple as this. It's just the same procedure as reading food labels, although you need to figure out the portion size by yourself (which is why we use a food scale). If you know the number of calories per 100 g. that your food choice contains, you can use the food scale and simple multiplication to calculate your calories.

Let's use one more example to further illustrate how simple calorie counting with a food scale is. For this example, you'll be eating two apples. A simple Google search reveals that apples contain 52 calories per 100 g. When you weigh the two apples the scale shows 372 g. Let's do the math:

> ➤ *3.72 × 52 = 193.44 calories*

The above math is completely accurate today, and it will be accurate tomorrow as well. Hence, when you eat apples of a comparable size in the future, knowing what you now know, you could just as well do the math in your head. One apple is roughly 100 calories, and two apples is roughly 200 calories. As you might notice, if you have a decent memory, you only need to use the food scale once or twice to know how many calories a particular meal contains.

If you consume entities of food that are relatively constant, for example apples and eggs, you can safely do the math in your head. The key is that you use *common sense*. Don't use head math when you eat a bowl of ice cream, because 'a bowl' could be of any size. But if it's an ice cream on a stick and you've already measured it once, then for sure use head math! As long as the amount of what you're eating is static, you can be safe about the accuracy of the calorie content.

When you're unsure of the calorie contents of something, or when the food label alone can't help you, *always* use your food scale. The most important thing is that you're *accurate* when tracking your calories. As long as you use common sense, you're fine. If ever unsure, rely on your friend, the food scale, instead of your guesstimations.

Method #3: Using a Fitness App

This third method is only recommended for certain situations. When we're not able to weigh our food, see any food labels, or use head math, fitness apps can be helpful and give us a decent estimation of the number of calories we're likely to consume. Here's an example of the situation I'm referring to: you're invited to eat at a restaurant with friends and family. Since you can't find the nutritional value/contents online (which many franchises and restaurants have started to provide), you'll have to estimate an approximate calorie amount. Let's say your plate looks like this:

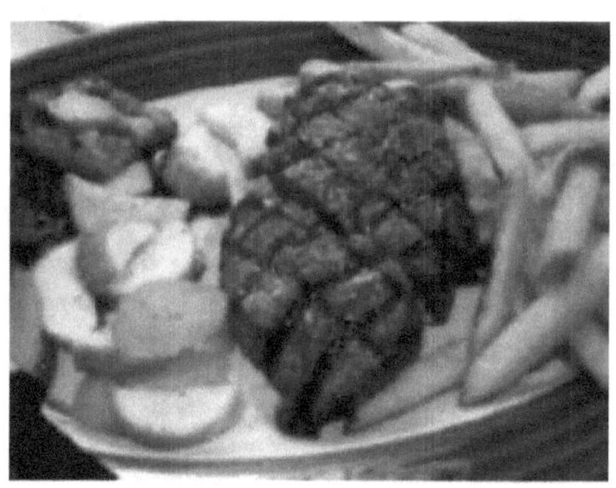

You're likely to know what type of meat you're eating (ribeye in this case), which is useful information. If you're lucky, you also have a clue about the size of the steak. This is something you can ask the waiter or may even find on the menu. Regardless, let's estimate the steak to be around 250 g. for the sake of this example, and use a fitness app to find out how many calories a ribeye steak contains per 100 g.

Calories in Ribeye

Nutrition Facts

Generic - Ribeye

Servings: 100.0 | 1 g

Calories	291	Sodium	54 mg
Total Fat	22 g	Potassium	260 mg
Saturated	10 g	Total Carbs	0 g
Polyunsaturated	1 g	Dietary Fiber	0 g
Monounsaturated	11 g	Sugars	0 g
Trans	1 g	Protein	24 g
Cholesterol	80 mg		
Vitamin A	0%	Calcium	1%
Vitamin C	0%	Iron	12%

*Percent Daily Values are based on a 2000 calorie diet. Your daily values may be higher or lower depending on your calorie needs.

If a ribeye steak contains 291 calories per 100 g., and you've ordered a 250 g. steak, the simple math is this:

> ➢ *2.5 × 291 = 727.50 calories*

The first part is now done. Let's continue using the same app. This time we'll estimate how many grams of fries you'll be consuming. Information about the portion size of the fries isn't as readily available as the information about the steak size. Such information is just not common, so you need to estimate the weight by yourself, then go on to use the fitness app to find a representative caloric value. This is what one result for French fries (out of roughly 20,000) reveals:

Calories in French Fries (Grams)

Nutrition Facts

Generic - French Fries (Grams)

Servings: 1.0	100 g		
Calories	140	Sodium	260 mg
Total Fat	14 g	Potassium	0 mg
Saturated	3 g	Total Carbs	2 g
Polyunsaturated	0 g	Dietary Fiber	0 g
Monounsaturated	0 g	Sugars	1 g
Trans	0 g	Protein	1 g
Cholesterol	10 mg		
Vitamin A	0%	Calcium	0%
Vitamin C	2%	Iron	0%

*Percent Daily Values are based on a 2000 calorie diet. Your daily values may be higher or lower depending on your calorie needs.

If we estimate there's about 200 g. of fries on the plate, here's the math:

> ➢ *2 × 140 = 280 calories*

Now we have the calories for the steak and the fries down. Naturally, we also need to add up the salad, any sauce, and any calorie-containing drink in the same way. For the sake of simplifying this example, we'll skip a few redundant steps and go straight to the finale. Let's add up all the caloric amounts we've estimated with help from our fitness app of choice and see what the total amount is.

> *Ribeye steak: 727.50 calories*

> *Fries: 280 calories*

> *Ketchup: 102 calories*

> *Salad: 77 calories*

> *Two pints of beer: 466 calories*

> ***Total number of calories: 1652.50***

As you'll have noted during the course of this example, this method is far less accurate than the food label and food scale ones, while simultaneously being far more complicated and time-consuming. However, as long as dinner with friends/family is an exception to your normal routine, the hassle won't bother you much.

In summary, just keep in mind that you want to avoid guesstimation as much as possible. You'll do better the simpler you keep things, which you'll soon learn more about in coming chapters. For now, know that 'KISS' (keep it simple, stupid) is no joke. Rather, it's one of the greatest principles you'll ever come across. Let simplicity guide you.

The Finale: Adding Up Your Total

This is what we've been after all along: the total number of calories you've consumed throughout the day. *How come?* The following lessons will treat precisely that question but, in essence, we simply want to collect data about your body. This data gives us the information we need to be able to transform. There are two pieces of data we need to collect on a daily basis, and your total daily intake of calories is one of them. There will be more on this in coming chapters, however. For now, we need to learn how to add up the total.

You probably already have a good idea about how this final calculation is to be made. We'll take no risks, however. Calorie counting should be so simple that even a five-year-old could learn it. So, for the sake of clarity, let's go through the final process together.

For this final example we'll say that you ate some of the exemplified meals from methods 1, 2, and 3 outlined earlier in this chapter. For simplicity's sake, we'll stick with the bland meals used earlier, even though they may be poor representations of actual breakfast/lunch/dinner meals. I appreciate the fact that few people actually eat plain rice for lunch, but please bear with me for clarity's sake. So, here's what we ate during the day:

- **A quick breakfast:** An apple and a protein bar
- **Normal lunch:** 141 g. of rice
- **Dinner with the family:** Steak and fries, plus two beers

Of course, all we need to do is add up the total number of calories consumed. If broken down, here's what the math would look like:

> *Apple: 96.72 calories*

- ➢ *Protein bar: 320 calories*
- ➢ *Rice: 521.70 calories*
- ➢ *Steak, fries, and beers: 1652.50 calories*
- ➢ **Total calories = 2590.92**

Now, how would the process of 'adding up' work in real life? We would document the calories in our phones directly after consuming them. I suggest you use your smartphone's calculator to do this. It's by far the simplest way to do it in my experience. All you need to do is add calories to your calculator as the day passes. This would mean that your calculator said this during the day:

After breakfast	After lunch	After dinner

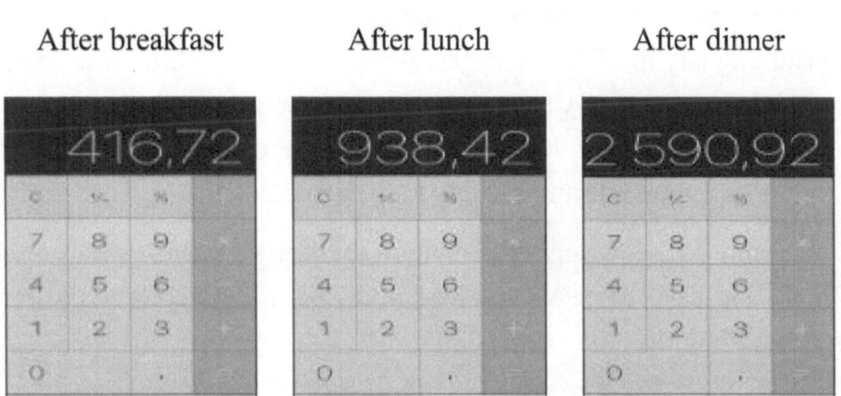

In case you need to use your calculator for something else, just screenshot the current amount you've added up, and put it back once you're done with the other calculation. It really is as simple as this. Just add up your calories using your phone's calculator. As I said, KISS.

Measurement and Documentation

It might sound intimidating, but you're going to be expected to engage in the practice of 'documentation' during Part 2. Really though, don't worry about it because it's incredibly simple. In essence, you're going to be tasked with tracking and documenting two factors on a daily basis, nothing else. It really is as simple as that.

These are the two factors you'll be tracking daily:

1. In the morning: your body weight
2. At night, before bed: your total calorie intake

In the mornings, weigh yourself after your toilet visits and before consuming any food or beverages. Just step on the bathroom scale and note the date and the weight in a document on your smartphone. At night, before going to bed, just make a note of the total number of calories consumed during the day in the same document. That's it.

Keeping notes is supposed to be simple and easy, and I mean *super* simple and easy. Here's what it should look like (a screenshot from my own phone):

18 apr
Weight: 91,3 kg
Kcal: 2267

19 apr
Weight: 91,4 kg
Kcal: 2321

20 apr
Weight: 91,2 kg
Kcal: 2198

21 apr
Weight: 91,0 kg
Kcal: 2177

22 apr
Weight: 90,8 kg
Kcal: 2251

See? This type of note will take less than a minute of your time each day. Measuring your weight and calorie intake is the most valuable habit you could practice, because the act of measurement is what ultimately gives you control over your body.

Here's what I mean. When you habitually collect factual information about how your body works, you'll soon be able to see trends; for example, x number of calories leads to more weight over time. Is the trend desired or not? With factual evidence at hand, you can manipulate your parameters, thus adjusting your body's trends in any direction you want. In other words, you'll be able to control your body's appearance any way you want.

In Preparation for Part 2

It's about time to get on with the more practical part of the book— 'the program,' if you will. It's basically a ten-week journey where you start learning how to practice the skill of transforming (maybe for the very first time). Part 2 is to be used in a very specific way, and it's tremendously important that it's used as intended.

The key rule is this: you're *not* to read further than the prevailing week. Although you're encouraged to revisit Part 1, as well as the current and all previous weeks, you're never intended to read 'ahead of time.' *Do* revisit the calorie counting chapters if necessary. *Do* go back and re-read the chapter about body fat, etc. Repetition is as welcome as it is useful. *It's absolutely essential*, however, that you consume Part 2 during a ten-week period (or longer if you require it). Hopefully, the importance of this one rule (which applies to Part 3 as well) is stated thoroughly enough.

Now: throughout the weeks, you'll get active and really start pursuing your ideal body. The journey will have its ups and downs, and it might feel awkward at times. For this reason, many get the urge to change up the process for various reasons, but this is what you ultimately want to avoid doing. That's why many of the ideas and mantras that may have already been mentioned will be repeated throughout Part 2.

Understanding patience will feel a hell of a lot different when you've been doing everything you should for a few weeks in a row, and you suddenly start seeing smaller and smaller results of weight loss. That's when you need to remember that weight loss isn't static. That's also when you need to remember that a few grams might not be a lot right now, but that a few grams over many months and years add up to a mountain of weight that you've lost. When things are tough, or when you're highly motivated, come back to Part 1 and Part 2 and remind yourself about the skill you're learning, and what type of journey you're on.

Part 2 includes several invitations for you to reflect, and is, in its nature, more of an epistolary text than Part 1. Many of the chapters in Part 2 were written when I was out in the field myself, transforming for the sake of reminding myself of how it feels so that I can better relay the experience to you, the reader. One short chapter often represents what I did or thought about during a full day on my own journey and, if you want to, you can use the chapters in the same way.

Before starting Part 2, I want to remind you that you're an individual. Understanding yourself and your own personality is what eventually will give you results. Anyone can be on a specific program for a period of time, but only if the program fits your personality will it be worthwhile for you to stay with it for longer. You're in charge of your journey, and you can make it into exactly what you want! As long as you're mindful about what you do, collect and document your personal data, and remain patient, you'll get there.

How you choose to go about meeting your calorie target, etc., is up to you. Remember that transforming is a skill that will last you a lifetime. If you create a go-to behavior and a go-to (sustainable) lifestyle that you can choose to adopt at one time or another, you have complete control over your body, and your ideal physique is always obtainable. It's a transformation away, and it's up to you to decide when you want to look a certain way.

I hope that repeating the following parable will help you mentally frame what you'll be doing over the coming weeks: give a man a fish and he will eat for a day; teach a man how to fish and you feed him for a lifetime.

By learning, once and for all, about your food behavior and how to track calories, you'll learn 'how to fish.' You *will* have to spend a bit of time and energy at first, because these skills don't come automatically. You most likely have to be willing to invest the effort for a few weeks, even if you struggle at first. You *will* have the abilities down eventually, however, and you *will* then have them down for life, just like you already can ride a bike.

Learning how to help yourself in this manner is a priceless investment, and you should see it as nothing less than that. Just try to imagine how a version of yourself with more energy and confidence would act at work and in social settings. The version of yourself that you can become is possible if you make the investment. I think Warren Buffett's take on investing in oneself is superb, and I'd like to share it here to further drive home the point and value of making an investment in yourself by taking charge of your body.

Warren Buffett has been judged the richest person in the world many times. This is as much due to his ability to invest in the *right people* as it is investing in the right businesses. He's often considered to be the best investor in history, and here's one of his fundamental lessons:

Again, just imagine how your performance at work would be affected by a more confident and energetic you. How would your social life change? Once you spend the energy to learn how you should behave in relation to food, you can forevermore decide what you want to look like. Once your food behavior is constructed by yourself in accordance with your goals, you can just switch the mode back to autopilot. Imagine being able to do the right thing without thinking—it's truly priceless. As I said, it's very possible. You only need to learn this once, before going back to autopilot.

When you feel ready, I'll see you in Part 2.

Part 2

THE TEN WEEK JOURNEY

Your Mental Investment

The act of doing is very different from the act of reading, listening, watching, or e-learning. Within the context of this part of the book, to be very clear, the *doing* is more important than anything else. Therefore, as soon as possible after starting this part of the journey, I want to urge you, dear reader, to make sure that you have all the necessary tools to hand. The tools are *absolutely essential*, and you can get them in a matter of minutes by, for example, purchasing them from a website of your choice. These things are extremely cheap, and they'll last you for many years to come, so don't worry about the initial investment. You can use any brand at any price as long as they work consistently. What you need is:

- An ordinary bathroom scale
- A food/kitchen scale
- A smartphone

If you're unable to get out of the house at this very moment, just get them from websites such as Amazon, or send out a text asking family members or friends if you can borrow theirs. Remember, it's the *doing*.

The principles and tasks outlined in this book are super simple but practicing them just isn't to start with. However, you'll learn the ropes in a matter of a few weeks. In this part, we'll go through the few weight loss strategies and principles that actually work, and your main challenge is to utilize those strategies and principles in practice until they become habitual.

The act of practicing is what separates those who get results from those who don't. Just think about it like this: if the principles are so simple, why doesn't everyone look the way they want? It's because most everyone doesn't practice what they know.

The key to your transformation success is making the practicing of the right principles habitual. Developing a new habit is said to take sixty-six days (just about ten weeks, like the length of the journey we're now on), according to Phillippa Lally, a health psychology researcher at University College London, and that's the challenge you should mentally prepare to conquer.

The best way to prepare is to develop your mental framework in advance. There will be ups and downs along your journey but, if you're prepared for these, you'll conquer each day with certainty. The mental framework I suggest you adopt, which is the same mental framework that I've used several times in my own attempts to transform, is as follows:

You're preparing to partake in a challenge that you have the means to conquer. You'll only be tasked with objectives you can successfully manage. Your mission is to practice the theoretical things you'll learn here. The investment you should mentally prepare for is a ten-week, self-enhancing experiment intended to develop great new habits. Prepare to act, to do things you're able to do, for a ten-week period.

That's all there is to it. You *can* do it, and you *will* do it, essentially. If you succeed with habituating the principles taught here, the processes outlined in this book will go from being simple in theory to being easy in practice, and you'll start to become a master of your own body.

These ten weeks have the potential to change your life forever. The practical knowledge you're teaching yourself from this book, the knowledge and skill to act with the right principles in mind, will give you a lifetime of control over your body. Give yourself this gift. Prepare to transform both physically and mentally over the next ten weeks.

Document the Starting Point

First of all, before starting the actual program, there are two more important things that need to be taken care of. First, you need to document the status quo. This means that you're to take some photos of yourself from a few different angles:

- From the front
- From one side
- From the back
- From the other side

These pictures are intended for your own purposes and you don't need to show them to anyone else. Selfies thus work just as well as normal photos. However, keep in mind that these photos will be used as comparisons with your future progress photos, so either use your camera's date facility or hold a newspaper or something similar to date the photos. If you have the slightest hunch that you'll want to show your progress to someone in the future, you'll want to date the photos.

Second, find a picture of a physique you admire and store it somewhere you very often get to see it (perhaps you can make it into your phone's background). There's one important caveat, however. You must choose a physique that you think you can achieve if you work diligently at it for about a year. And don't worry if this first target isn't your ideal body. You'll be able to aim higher and higher as you progress over time. What's important is that you have a fixed and achievable target, because once you reach it, you'll realize that you're in full control of your own body, and it's a wonderful experience.

As mentioned about 'doing' earlier, get those photos taken today. It only takes a few minutes.

Week 1
'How Are You Eating?'

Summary of what you'll be doing

- Tracking your calories on your smartphone on a daily basis.

- Documenting your weight every morning.

- Documenting your total calories every evening.

- Actively reflecting on your eating behavior.

Extra important during this week

- Do NOT change your normal food behavior.

- DO spend the extra time it takes to count and track your calories and weight. You're learning a new skill, so don´t worry if it feels awkward at first.

- If you struggle with remembering to document your numbers, set regularly occurring alarms on your phone to remind you. Do NOT miss the documentation.

During the first week of your journey, you're to track your calories and reflect about your food choices, but you're not yet to change any of your eating habits. This is very important. You'll spend the first week just tracking what you're doing—your eating behavior.

You'll realize one or two things about how your autopilot is set up just by tracking your behavior and calories. Make sure to be accurate and to document your weight and total calories by the end of the day, and you're golden.

We'll be able to work more actively with food choices, exercise, and calorie manipulation as time goes by. During the first week, however, you shouldn't change a single thing from what you normally do. Just be honest about the calories you consume (there's no judgment, regardless of what the current situation looks like).

As you go about the practical aspect of counting calories and putting the number into your phone's calculator, it's essential you also try to reflect as much as possible about what calories you've put into your system and why. Reflection is very much a forgotten activity, but it's a piece of gold that's very conducive to mental clarity and embedding new knowledge in your brain.

One thing I would want you to reflect upon is how aware you've been about what you were eating previously in your life, and what it feels like to see the caloric value of a food choice. While you add up calories, think about whether you've understood how many or how few calories you habitually consume without thinking. Imagine what you would look like if your habits were different.

After a few days, you should start to see patterns in your eating. Perhaps you eat a similar number of calories each day, or perhaps you're very volatile. The patterns you perceive may reveal much about your current food behavior, and maybe even some causes for it. If you find that 'high' and 'low' days (in terms of calorie consumption) appear randomly, it could be very productive to dig deeper into potential reasons for this. For instance, do you remember being stressed out on days of high calorie intake? What do you remember about the days of low intake?

You don't need to journal your thoughts or write them down anywhere, just ponder. Get to know yourself a little more. What you find out when reflecting upon these questions is how your daily life affects your eating. Eating is often preceded and followed by emotion, and very many people eat tasty and calorie-dense food to curb stress. Good food soothes, but only for the short term. Since too much good food can't be undone, anxiety can often follow. More food may then dampen the anxiety. Isn't it obvious why it's easy to become addicted to good food?

Thinking About Food

Do a quick Google-search on the following words before you read on: what does 200 calories look like?

Once you've had a look, have a think about the following question: what do you think would fill you up more, 740 g. of mini peppers or 100 g. of peanut butter?

This is actually a trick question, and as the weeks go on, you'll learn a whole lot more about why such and similar questions are the wrong ones to ask. If we don't like mini peppers, it becomes irrelevant whether they would hypothetically fill us up more than peanut butter (or an equivalent calorie-dense food we really enjoy). We wouldn't eat the mini peppers (at least not on a daily basis for years to come, and not instead of peanut butter during all this time), and that's an issue.

The hypothetical mini pepper situation is what I think is one of the biggest issues with health, fitness, and appearance advice in general. A theoretical argument doesn't automatically transfer well into reality. Arguing for a vegetable-filled diet, abstinence from fast food, alcohol, etc., is very logical from an intellectual and theoretical perspective. I'm sure this is something you already understand. What's missing is the guidance that helps us to become self-sufficient. You must learn the skills and abilities that help you construct enjoyable and sustainable habits that lead to desired results.

Arguing from a purely logical perspective is as productive as arguing that people should invest several thousand dollars in the stock market monthly, because more is more is better, right? No, not everyone has thousands to spare, and even if they did, what's right still depends on each person's individual situation, tax bracket, risk tolerance, etc. Being logical isn't the way to go, at least not for our intents and purposes. We need to be pragmatic. That's what we are becoming in this book.

The Weekend

As the week progresses, you'll inevitably experience the weekend, regardless of what day it was when you started counting calories. This is an interesting period, because the absolute majority of people I've met have a different routine during weekends compared to weekdays. What you tend to do on weekends is very important information, so keep tracking your calorie intake, and don't neglect anything. By this I mean that alcohol, fast food, coffee drinks—everything—is to be accounted for as accurately as possible. Again, we're striving to understand your food behavior *as it is.*

You can't be right or wrong in your food behavior, and there's nothing to be ashamed of, regardless of what it is you consume. We simply need to understand what's going on.

I know that this is repetitive, but rest assured this will be repeated many times more. Tracking your calories and understanding your food behavior is key. If you learn how to achieve an understanding about yourself, being honest and accurate, you're set for life.

Preparation for Next Week

As you may have noticed, immense activity and drastic life changes aren't the keys to achieving a transformation. Knowledge and understanding about yourself, derived from tracking your calories and weight, and from reflecting upon your food behavior, is what *actually* brings about results. This is so because eventually we'll know how many calories we need to move our weight in a desired direction.

Once we understand why we're where we're at, we can start adjusting a few things (and you'll know when it's time for this; it's not right now). In the beginning, the smallest changes will make a huge difference, and your lifestyle will likely have to change very little. As we get further along, however, the progress will likely require a bit more. That's when we start replacing certain food choices and habits with other habits, to maintain as much of our lifestyles as possible.

The word 'lifestyle' is truly important. A common issue I see a lot is that people try to remove anything remotely associated with the words 'bad' or 'unhealthy' (perhaps 'fun' is a good synonym). The most successful people in terms of the endeavor you're pursuing, however, instead learn to replace old habits and foods with potent variations that fulfill the same purposes (being emotionally and physically filling, tasty, fun, pleasurable, etc.), but with fewer side effects (weight gain, anxiety, social sacrifice, etc.).

This is what we eventually want to do, so that we not only can achieve a new body, but also maintain it. Most of the people who have been successful in the short term and, especially, the long term, have replaced old habits while still deriving the same value and pleasure they used to experience as a result of the old lifestyle. Imagine being able to enjoy your life while also achieving your ideal body—this is what we want to strive for (patiently).

What to Expect During Next Week

In the second week, we'll start making very minute adjustments that steer you in the direction of the scenario just described, where you live an enjoyable lifestyle while still reaching your goals. You will *not* be asked to worry about how much you eat, or where the calories come from. In this sense, weeks 1 and 2 are identical. However, you *will* be asked to complete *one* important task, which is to make *one* conscious food choice during the week—just one. The goal is to find a way to make one of your food choices during the week less calorically dense. There will be more about the task in the next chapter.

Week 2
Still, 'How Are You Eating?'

Summary of what you'll be doing

- Tracking your calories on your smartphone on a daily basis.

- Documenting your weight every morning.

- Documenting your total calories every evening.

- **Task:** Make *one* conscious food choice at some point during the week.

Extra important during this week

- Do NOT change your normal food behavior.

- Keep reflecting and remain patient.

Although once you're into the second week, it's technically the eighth day of your journey, I suggest you view every week as a new week, and every individual day as a new day. Taking each day at a time is a very smart strategy, not just for short-term results, but specifically for long-term ones.

Getting results isn't a matter of perfection, which is a common false belief. Results come from doing the right things more often than doing the wrong things over a period of time. In other words, it's about maintaining a trend. Naturally, you would make things easier for yourself if you did 'the right things' more frequently, but don't take this sentiment the wrong way. I don't say it's easier because results would come much quicker (they won't), but I say this because doing the right thing more frequently leads to routine, which in turn makes it easier for you to stay consistent.

Consistently doing the right thing, at least more often than you do the wrong thing, leads to results. It's as simple as that: our struggle is to stay consistent. So, how do we go about that?

There's no one answer to the above question. Here's something to keep in mind, however. Everyone can track food and body weight for one day. Everyone can do it for a week too. The same reasoning is usually what helps people who struggle with far more challenging tasks than ours; for example, overcoming addiction. They take one day at a time. In small enough pieces, it's possible to handle most anything.

So, while there are many ways to remain consistent with a lifestyle that's worthwhile, whether that's a sober, virtuous, or healthy one, splitting up the parts of your life that challenge you into smaller parts that are manageable is probably one of the greater methods in terms of efficiency, simplicity, and longevity.

Your Task This Week

During *one* meal of your choice, you're to make a conscious food choice. The point of the exercise is *not* to replace your lunchtime pasta for a salad, or anything similar to that. The idea is that you consciously reflect about what you're in the mood for, and how you can make that choice as calorically light as possible.

Some people realize that they can remove 140 calories from their meal by replacing their regular 330 ml. can of Coke with a no-calorie variant or water. Others have realized that they can order a pasta ragu instead of a carbonara and save hundreds of calories.

Simply, your task is to make *one* of these conscious food choices during the week. The sole goal is to find out how you can achieve the same life experience you urged for, with fewer calories spent.

Preparation for Next Week

By now, you have two weeks' data. What I would like you to do is figure out what your average calorie intake is. Add up the fourteen different daily totals you've submitted in your document and divide the sum by fourteen.

I've seen diverse calorie averages over the years, but they rarely go far outside of the 2,000–5,000 range. Whatever your average is, round it down to a nice even number (the closest hundred). This means that if you, for instance, consumed an average of 3,092.8 calories during the first two weeks, you would round it down to 3,000.

Your caloric average, whatever it is, is your new, daily calorie target for the entirety of next week! The goal in the upcoming week is to consume *no more* and *no less* than those 3,000 (for example) calories. It doesn't matter if you're full or not, you're to meet your target anyway.

Week 3
Controlling What You Eat

Summary of what you'll be doing

- Remaining consistent with a set caloric target.

- Tracking your calories on your smartphone on a daily basis.

- Documenting your weight every morning.

- Documenting your total calories every evening.

- **Task:** Create a ritual.

Extra important during this week

- Calculate your daily calorie target and adhere to it (within +/- 50 calories is okay).

- Do NOT stop eating if you're full and have calories left to consume.

- STOP eating if you don't have any calories left to consume, even if you're hungry.

This week, we're really starting to get into the real stuff. Likely, if you've never had a fixed caloric target to hit consistently, this week might feel a bit unusual and/or awkward. Hopefully, however, this is a period during which your confidence and motivation is at its highest, so hopefully the oddness of the journey will feel more like a fun experiment than a burdensome chore.

You've just come off two weeks where hunger hasn't been an issue, while you've simultaneously learned to practice the skill of calorie counting. This means that progress has already been made, and that you're already on your way to your ideal physique. If you could remain consistent with counting calories and documenting your weight and daily calories during the first two weeks, you've proven to yourself that you can complete this week too … remember this.

The only difference between this week and the prior ones is that it's mandatory to be conscious about your food behavior all the time. This is because you have a caloric target that you need to hit on a daily basis, and if you don't make sure to consciously budget your calories, you won't be able to remain consistent with this target. Simple as that.

This is the first week during which you might have to face the emotion of hunger or the sensation of being very full, but still having to consume another few hundred calories. These are the moments where *you* need to step up and make the executive decisions, not allow your emotions or old habits to make those decisions. Hitting your caloric target is priority number one. Your day revolves around this goal.

Routine

Now that you've gotten this far into your journey, it's important to delve a bit deeper into the topic of routine. How does tracking your calories and weight feel after roughly two weeks of practicing these habits? Have a think about it. An indicator that things are heading in the right direction for you is that the task of tracking starts to feel easier and easier. Such a trend indicates that your new habits are starting to form, and that you're developing the type of behavior that gives you control over your body.

If things aren't starting to feel easier, then something isn't working as it should, and we need to troubleshoot. The most common issue, I've found, is a turbulent lifestyle. The less daily routine, the harder it is to achieve consistency. Having to adjust to new challenges on a daily basis takes mental energy, for one. If you're spent, mentally, your likelihood of saying 'fuck it' increases significantly. Second, the mere lack of a set routine in itself makes it more difficult to form a new habit. If you can't choose to repeat a successful day, you constantly have to reinvent different versions of successful days. This works too but takes a significantly longer time. Many confuse themselves in this area. A person who isn't successful from the start isn't untalented, just human.

We fail, we learn, and try again, stronger and wiser. That's one of the main points of life! People who, for various reasons, be it work, family, life-related, or something else, struggle with developing sturdy routines to follow on a daily basis, have a tougher challenge to conquer than their opposites. They're *not* weaker or less talented, although too many seem to believe such falsehoods. My suggestion is to take it for what it is.

People with different circumstances have different challenges to tackle. Some will have an easier time by default, and there's nothing we can do to change that. We can only try to embrace and appreciate the lot we've been given. Believe it or not, all personal lots carry benefits and downsides. Try to find at least one benefit of having your own lot. My personal favorite, being a person who struggles with getting lean, is that I have an easier time packing on muscle. So, from now on, start trying to think about your strengths.

Your Task This Week

One of the most effective strategies for building routine, at least that I've found over the years, is the utilization of rituals. How is a ritual defined in this context? A ritual is an activity that's performed regularly—optimally daily—for a set period of time. This could be a vow to drink a large glass of water before eating dinner every day.

The point of such a ritual, which I've used for brief periods of time, is twofold. First, if you're lucky, that large glass of water may help you eat a little less food during the coming sitting. However, the effect itself is minuscule, even at best, but that's not the point. The most important part is the second point, which is solidifying of your goal via action. The activity of drinking a glass of water before dinner, regardless of the effectiveness of such a procedure, is in alignment with your goal to eat with a caloric target in mind, and you solidify this goal to yourself with a memorable activity. Not only will it help guide your thoughts and solidify your behavior, it makes you feel good about yourself too. It makes you feel like you're actually doing it!

A ritual can be many things, and I have a few that I depend on during different stages of my body transformation. Various health supplements can be used in place of the water, for instance. Their actual benefit isn't the point, but the behavior that you're solidifying is.

However, there are two major points to consider with rituals:

1. Avoid the common trap of overdoing. A ritual is a routine-building, behavioral strategy. It takes time, patience, and repetition. It's not a shortcut or a pill. The actual health/transformative benefits from the things you choose to do are minuscule. The behavior is the key. So, use rituals with caution, and don't overconsume either water or a supplement.

2. Set a time limit to the ritual, otherwise you may get backlash. Adhering to a ritual that's in alignment with your goals should be a sound and positive aspect of your life. Promising yourself to adhere to a ritual, no matter how sound it is, for life, is unnecessary. If you make a lifetime commitment, even a single slip from the ritual may result in feelings of remorse and anxiety. Rituals constitute small details in the grand scheme of what produces positive results. Having more good days than bad is what will eventually get you there. Slipping on a small detail like a ritual isn't a big deal. Following a ritual for a period of six to eight weeks is often very beneficial, however.

Create a ritual for yourself and see if it doesn't remind you about the fact that you're making progress. Rituals should be easy and safe, and preferably also mentally satisfying. Starting the day off with a cup of black coffee, determined not to eat until lunchtime, is a ritual I established years ago, and whenever I start getting serious about transforming into a slimmer version, I go back to it for a period of time. You'll learn more about this and about 'how to not eat' as we go along. Eventually, you'll make up your own strategies that do the same trick for you too. The point is that a good ritual can take you far.

Preparation for Next Week

This week has been all about remaining consistent with your caloric target and taking control of your food behavior. In the coming week, control will be paired with manipulation too. Not only will you keep practicing your conscious food behavior and calorie/weight tracking, but you'll also learn how to manipulate your calories to steer your body in your desired direction.

For next week, you're to subtract 100 calories from your daily target and adhere to the new target. To help overcome any potential hunger-related issue that stems from the controlled eating behavior, we'll introduce a practical task that makes it more difficult for you to feel hungry. More on this in the coming chapter of your journey.

Week 4
Control and Manipulate

Summary of what you'll be doing

- Remaining consistent with your *new* caloric target (100 calories less).

- Tracking your calories on your smartphone on a daily basis.

- Documenting your weight every morning.

- Documenting your total calories every evening.

- **Task:** Take pictures.

Extra important during this week

- Manage your hunger and emotions. Do NOT give into your hunger. Try to appreciate the journey and be happy instead.

You Will Not Die

Given that you have fewer calories to play around with this week, we need to put a few things into perspective. One thing I say to all who are serious about their transformation is this: 'you *will* not die.' The context? Hunger. And, usually, the statement arises from a practical experiment that I have some do. Many have never spent a single day of their lives without eating, not a single one. The thing is that the body is more resilient than one might think. Going without food for twenty-four hours is more of a mental struggle than a physical one. Therefore, I urge some people to go a full day without eating (but not you, not right now).

There's a second context to the statement too, and it's a bit harsher. At times, we all just need to quiet down and accept the fact that we live in a beautiful world at a wonderful time. Being hungry or, rather, feeling hungry once or twice a day for one or two hours is *not* an issue. Not at all. Often, it's the opposite of an issue. Hunger is very habitual, and if we feel hunger frequently, and if we also have excess weight that we can transform away, we're part of the richest percentile in the world. First of all, that means that we should be appreciative of the fact we don't have to worry about food. Second, we have enough of a social safety net to ensure we won't starve to death very easily. You *will* not die.

Rest assured that this (hunger) too shall pass. Trust yourself—you're stronger than you think. With good enough reasons, you can do remarkable things in this world. A little hunger is nothing to you. Be proud of the fact that you're willing to learn something new—the skill of transformation—and simply plug along. You'll get to your goal, and things like hunger and other speedbumps will become easier and easier to handle the more used to the process you get.

Reasons

Building upon the idea of 'good enough reasons,' please reflect on the following concept for a minute: do it for someone else. There are a lot of ways and areas that 'doing it for someone else' can be applied to achieve results. Start by imagining that a doctor lets you know you're at risk of a heart attack due to certain life choices. How would your family react? Maybe your parents have to experience the fear that they'll outlive their child. Such and similar horrors never just affect one person. The positive and negative life choices we make have the chance to affect people around us. You should therefore also try to imagine an opposite scenario. What if you were that person that turned their life around? How would your partner feel about a you that suddenly has more energy and confidence due to smarter food and life choices? Even more, how would they feel if your appearance suddenly started to change for the better too?

I always think this is a useful thought to play around with. You could make your family and partner very happy just by taking care of yourself. Wouldn't you be happy if the reverse happened to you? It would be like receiving a gift, a gift that's impossible to purchase. If you choose to make positive changes in your life for someone else, you have the ability to give this as a gift to someone of your choice. You get all the pleasure from feeling the accomplishment, but you, more importantly, get the true reward, the gift of giving something of real value to someone else. Do it for someone you want to give everything to. Be the person you wish entered your own life.

Repetition, Repetition

I've already mentioned that most of the things that are explained in this book are different renditions of similar concepts. Listening and trying to grasp what's said may almost feel like repetitive brainwashing, and that, funnily enough, is part of the objective. A transformation journey is something that takes day-to-day action and thought. A successful transformation requires the repetition of 'good days' as it's the only way I've seen people succeed and be able to keep up their results.

Having one 'good day' after the other; that is, 'having a target number of calories and pursuing it by utilizing individualized tactics that facilitate your consuming the right number of calories without sacrificing longevity or too much of your wellbeing, and repeating that same process day after day,' may seem like a bit of a tall task, especially when put this way–intentionally complex. However, it's really not once it's become habitual. That's why I regard transforming as a skill, and why routine is so damn important. Routine helps you achieve good days without even thinking, and that's when you have your autopilot set up the right way. When you routinely and automatically live through more and more 'good days,' results not only start appearing, but the paradigm of complexity soon forces itself out of your head too. Why think about a transformation in the complex way just exemplified? Instead, you can just 'repeat good days.' How simple, right?

Communicating and teaching the skill of transformation requires repetition and frequent guidance. An autopilot takes a bit of time and patience to achieve, but it's very, very achievable. Accept the task of learning the skill of transformation and accept it for the long term. As long as you put the effort into having good days, it will eventually become habitual, and finally as easy as it's simple. All you need are more good days than bad ones. Stay strong, stay on track, and repeat the good days.

Appreciation

Some of the best advice I ever received, which I now would like to pass on to everyone who aspires to transform, is this: make sure you try to appreciate the journey. Appreciation doesn't have to be esoteric or philosophical, that's not the intention here. Appreciation is the active effort you put into enjoying the lifestyle that comes with your goal. It's fun to be the boss of your own brain, and telling it when it's time to eat, not the other way around.

Appreciation is finding out how much less money you spend on food and alcohol for the duration of the transformation and taking pride in this important change. You could even be appreciative of the future pleasures you get to imagine: how good will it feel to take off your shirt at that pool party you've been waiting for and have a well-deserved beer? You'll be asked how a physique like yours is compatible with beer, how you did it, etc., and that feels great.

Appreciate this future reward. If you're really successful with your transformation, you may even attract some envy and suddenly hear that you've had great genetics all along, which is interesting. It's one of the best types of compliment, so enjoy it!

I urge you to do your best to enjoy the journey for what it is. Enjoy the results you imagine, because if you keep tracking your calories and remain patient, you're well on your way there. It's a matter of a few months, take your time and appreciate it.

Your Task This Week

You've already documented your starting point and you may already have seen some results in the weight loss department. However, it isn't as certain that you've noticed significant changes in your appearance. This is why you're now to take some new pictures. As before, you want to snap a picture from the front, side, back, and other side. No one but you has to see them, and you take them for comparative reasons, so try to take the pictures in the same room as you did the first ones, using similar lighting, similar distance, etc.

What you may notice when comparing your starting photos with your new ones, are slight changes in some areas of your body. This may be the first time you realize that you've made some true progress, so really try hard to appreciate this. We often get so used to seeing ourselves that we fail to realize the slight changes that have taken place.

Since I was a child, I always thought I saw the same person in the mirror every day, even now when I'm twice as tall and three times as heavy. Only when I compare how I used to look do I realize what's been going on throughout the years. The point I'm trying to get at is don't fool yourself into thinking that you're not making progress because it's not blatantly obvious at this exact moment. You're making progress, and you'll get there. Just compare your pictures and see for yourself.

Preparation for Next Week

For the coming week, you're once more to remove 100 calories from your target. If you have the urge to remove even more, *don't*. Remember to be patient. The best thing you can do is to prepare mentally for another week of doing what you need to do. Boredom, weirdly enough, is a common foe when it comes to transformations.

After a few weeks, the urge to overdo usually sets in, and that's a major pipe dream. You can't shortcut the journey. For next week, you're simply to keep going, nothing else. Prepare mentally.

Week 5
Additional Manipulation and Control

Summary of what you'll be doing

- Remaining consistent with your *new* caloric target (another 100 calories less).

- Tracking your calories on your smartphone on a daily basis.

- Documenting your weight every morning.

- Documenting your total calories every evening.

- **Task:** Try out a 'golden' food.

- Learning about how to combat boredom and remaining patient.

Extra important during this week

- Do NOT get tricked into overdoing. You have a target—simply adhere to it.

Don't Overdo It

When trying to figure out how to transform on their own, or when trying to transform without a reasonable timeline as guidance, many people end up going on drastic programs for a few weeks, be it a crash diet, a magical supplement cycle, or an extreme exercise regime, which can be effective, but most often isn't. As you're well aware, you're only to remove 100 calories this week, no more.

Being drastic tends to be a finite solution to the process of transformation. Most struggle with adjusting to the drastic lifestyle changes such programs require, either because life's other obligations get in the way, or because the lifestyle changes themselves require too much energy to sustain. So, nothing is intrinsically wrong with any program, it's more an issue of compatibility. Most people shouldn't opt for the drastic programs because real-life obligations and decades of opposite habit building get in the way.

That's why I urge you to take it slow and steady, while having a long-term perspective. If you're making progress, you've nothing to worry about. Transforming takes time and consistency. Keep striving to meet your target calories for the day. Keep weighing yourself. You're getting there, bit by bit. More importantly, however, when adopting the long-term perspective, you're learning to stay where you want. Keeping the results for the long term is just as important as getting there in the first place.

A Slip-Up

Despite my constant nagging about not overdoing it, there's an opposite scenario to be wary of too. The opposite of overdoing it would be to give up control completely, either for a short period of time or altogether. The thing is, there may come a time when you consume something that wasn't planned and that causes you to go significantly over your calorie target. Whether it's a misread label or a moment where human instincts overtake control, it can happen to anyone. When something like this happens, you should start by forgiving yourself.

Giving in to instincts or making a mistake doesn't make a person weak or immoral. Most likely, the situation occurred because there was a need to be spontaneous, a need to react to circumstances. In such cases, it's very difficult to make the best choices, especially if you don't have years of experience to rely on. When emotions steer our behavior, they're not easy to override. Therefore, having a moment where something unplanned is consumed is likely to happen at one time or another.

This may lead to feelings of anxiety or regret, but you shouldn't let these emotions take a hold of you. As long as you accept what's happened and work on getting back on your plan, you've nothing to worry about! You'll keep improving as long as you dare to get back on your plan, time after time.

The pitfall you need to avoid is letting one unplanned meal turn into a negative spiral and an eventual complete loss of control. Experiencing a very human moment—reacting based on emotions and instincts—is natural. Getting back on the horse is difficult, but it's the right thing to do. As long as you commit to keep trying, to keep doing your best, you've nothing to worry about. Stay strong and learn from your experiences!

Your Task This Week

Slip-ups can happen to anyone, but there are means at our disposal that help reduce the number of such occurrences. 'Golden' foods is one such means. You're to be introduced to it by trying something practical. It's a simple task, but there are reasons behind it. First, the task:

- I want you to fit one bowl of oatmeal porridge (using between 80–150 g. of oatmeal) into your eating for the day. The objective is to eat the porridge at some time during the day, while staying within your target calories.

Why should you try this then? There are two main reasons. The first is that people generally satisfy their hunger with oatmeal. It's almost always a great food choice, and it's filling. The second reason is that I want to encourage you to experiment with food choices. No matter who you are as a person, there are golden food choices to be found. It just takes an individual's own thoughts and efforts to find them.

Oatmeal is a personal golden food, and it's a primary go-to food for me whenever I start the process of transformation, because it helps me stay on track and still enjoy myself. Anyone who has just two or three different golden foods will have all the tools needed to eat in perfect accordance with their plan during most of their days. Just imagine if you had two of your own golden foods to be your lunch and dinner. How easy would it be to stay on track then?

As I said, what constitutes a golden food will vary from person to person, so it will be somewhat of an effort finding the foods in the first place. The simplest way to scout for golden foods is to judge the food by certain criteria. The golden food should be:

- cheap

- nutritious

- low to moderate calories

- filling

- tasty

Plain, simple oatmeal porridge, just as it is, meets four out of the five listed criteria (it's cheap, nutritious, moderate calories, and filling). If I add a flavorful protein powder to my porridge, I can make it a five out of five. Oatmeal has helped me stay on track more days than I can count.

Golden foods do most of the work for you. All you have to worry about is eating until you're full. Once you're fully satisfied, you haven't compromised your caloric goal. Start experimenting for yourself. Once you've found your gold, your journey will become much, much simpler.

Combating Boredom—Take a Walk

It's time now for me to have the pleasure of introducing 'the walk,' which is by far my favorite method for combating boredom, distracting myself from hunger, and for enhancing my reflecting.

After a certain amount of time of being on a caloric deficit, something subtle tends to happen to many people—their focus and thoughts turn inward, and they become a bit more introspective than they've previously been. What tends to become more and more enjoyable in this state of mind are ideas and pure thought. This is why I often recommend audiobooks/podcasts and long walks after a certain period of time on a transformation journey. It's not only stimulating and satisfying mentally, but it's immensely effective health-wise too.

Walking is a type of activity most people can do consistently for a long period of time without burning out or getting injured. So, if you're thinking about starting to do cardio, I highly recommend you take a long walk alongside good music or a good book rather than go out running or do various forms of interval training. Walking, as opposed to most (pretty much *all*) other forms of more intensive cardiovascular activity, is enjoyable. Just to be clear, I want to emphasize that this is opinion and not fact. However, with our intents and purposes in mind, I also want to point out that walking is what's helped me and the people that I've come across the most. That's why I'm such a strong proponent of the walk.

Efficiency discussions aside, however, my main point is that the walk is so much more than cardio. It's a great distracter from boredom and hunger, and a great catalyst for thought and reflection. Although walks can (and soon enough will) be used as cardio and a minor weight loss assistance tool, I want it primarily to be considered a source of enjoyment and general wellbeing.

It's common for people to start looking forward to weekends consisting of long walks with many great books playing in their ears, and isn't that something? There's a tremendous difference in seeking quick stimulants, from food, alcohol, entertainment, etc., and wanting to seek mental clarity and calm. The introspective part of the transformation process is precious, and whenever I come upon it, I try to appreciate it fully.

If you stick with your target calories for long enough, you'll most likely get to the introspective part of the transformation too, eventually. Look for signs that it's arrived and ride the introspective wave.

Preparation for Next Week

You're to remain with the same calorie target during next week. Instead of manipulating your calories, we'll have a look at what you can do with the ones you have. For instance, 3,000 calories can feel a lot different depending on whether you need to consume them all at the same time, or whether they come from liquids, etc. There are various alternatives for you to consider. How you choose to use your calories is an important topic, and it will be our main focus during next week.

Week 6
Using Hunger Tactics and Understanding Consequences

Summary of what you'll be doing

- Remaining consistent with your caloric target (same as last week).

- Tracking your calories on your smartphone on a daily basis.

- Documenting your weight every morning.

- Documenting your total calories every evening.

- Learning about macronutrients and common sense.

- Reflecting about eating behavior and consequences.

Extra important during this week

- Reflection is *essential* during this week. Really think deeply about your eating behavior and try to adjust your behavior in a productive direction.

Far into the Process—Still the Same Principles

Good routines and habits are fundamental when it comes to taking control of your body. Since you started this book, you've started to create good new routines and habits when it comes to your eating behavior. That's enough for the coming months, so don't feel stressed about adding cardio or exercise just because it's been mentioned recently. You're doing fine if you just keep track of your calories, and I can't stress this enough. It's essential you don't get overwhelmed and think you need to change everything you know about life right away. For one, we won't change your caloric target this week, which is a bit of evidence for this. As always, stay patient. This journey is made one step at a time.

The order of priority for your journey is, and always has been, this: first, becoming mindful of *how* you eat, which we started learning during the first two weeks. Then, you start *controlling* your eating for eight weeks, which is what this and the following weeks are all about. It's really that simple, even if it takes many pages of text to explain it.

After ten weeks on this journey, we're going to be able to evaluate what needs to be done next to keep progressing. There's an entire separate part in the book about that stage of your continued journey, which we'll get to later, so don't worry about it right now. Until then, the intention is to *not* change more than necessary.

The most important part right now is that your eating stays under *your* control. Avoiding slip-ups and managing your hunger is essential if you're to remain in control and keep getting results. As I hinted at in the preparatory section regarding this week, there are many ways to consume calories. Eventually, remaining consistent with a calorie target can become more of a strain than it initially was. Usually, this tends to happen between weeks 4–7, I've found. This is why we're now focusing on various tactics to help you cope with and enjoy life, while still reaching your goals and transforming.

Naturally, if you've never tried these tactics, they might feel awkward. However, it's very possible to make these hunger tactics habitual. When you learn about these tactics, just try to imagine that they could be part of your new behavioral autopilot. Not only would you always have the means to look the way you want, but you would automatically be heading towards your goals too. This is when the process goes from being simple to being easy.

Hunger Tactics

As already mentioned, I've intentionally included this section at a point when you're well into this book as, hopefully, the featured tactics are more of a relief this far into the process than they would be if they were introduced during the first week.

A few weeks into the process, especially if it's your first time transforming, it becomes increasingly important to keep hunger at bay. The journey takes the time it takes, and your patience may start to be tested. As much as we would like to, there's nothing we can do about time. It passes by at its own pace. Consuming fewer calories than your target suggests or exercising more than is necessary is a detriment to the process. Patience and consistency are the only known medicine. However, it's possible to make the time a little more bearable.

This isn't magical. You won't be able to apply any of these tactics to affect your progress. However, since you've been combating hunger for a while, the relief from your struggle by means of different ways of consuming your calories will feel very tangible. It's almost like a placebo. There's no medicine, but you feel better. Use these tactics now to make the new lifestyle easier. Use them later to gain healthy weight when it's time for that again. The two tactics to use are intermittent fasting and what I call replacement.

Intermittent fasting has become very popular in the last few years. Many fitness influencers started spreading the word about it on YouTube close to a decade ago, and hereditary methods like the 5:2 Diet have since sprung up. The underlying idea of intermittent fasting is really simple, so for you to avoid any unnecessary confusion that might result from hearing about it from multiple sources, please just accept the following, very rudimentary but essentially very accurate explanation: intermittent fasting is about creating time windows during which you can eat. Simple. Some people choose to consume all their calories between 12 p.m. and 8 p.m., some use other timeframes. It's nothing fancy, and it can be completely arbitrary.

Do you want to eat all your calories between 5 p.m. and 9 p.m.? If so, go ahead. The point of it all is that you'll have a more difficult time consuming all of your daily calories when there's a deadline attached. A 2,000-calorie meal will fill most people up, and if that meal happens to be your first one of the day, and if the clock says 6 p.m., you're in a very good position to stay within your calorie target for the day.

I want to highlight two things about intermittent fasting that are key. First, you don't need to be very stoic to fast. If you just skip breakfast and make 8 p.m. your hard stop for the day, you'll easily achieve a fourteen-hour to sixteen-hour fast. Isn't that something? It may first appear crazy to even consider a sixteen-hour fast, but it's really very simple to achieve.

This brings me to the second point I would like to highlight: you eventually get very used to your timeframe, and you stop feeling hungry until it's time to eat. This is the best part. Imagine how much easier your life would be if you weren't hungry from breakfast until lunch, and then from lunch to dinner. The amount of willpower and energy you would have for other activities than managing your hunger would be enormous. That's the true power of intermittent fasting. When you have a rigid timeframe habitualized, it's truly like having an autopilot that steers you in the right direction. Not having to be hungry and knowing that you'll be able to eat a large meal a little bit later on that will actually satisfy you, gives you a sense of control. Being in control will also give you a sense of confidence.

If you have the means to control your hunger and decide when to eat, what's to stop you from succeeding with your transformation? Intermittent fasting can do this for you. Just know that it may take some time getting used to an eating window. In the beginning you're likely to feel hunger and question whether intermittent fasting is worth it. If you do get a timeframe down, however, you'll be able to reap the benefits just mentioned. This tactic might not be for everyone, but it's at least worth trying at one point in your life.

The second tactic I mentioned was replacement. It's a pretty obvious name for a tactic, and it's really not supposed to be more complicated than it first appears. The idea is simply to replace some of your favorite food choices with similar, lower calorie ones. Instead of eating ice cream, you eat frozen yoghurt, for example. It can't be overstated how important this tactic is. Everyone can intellectually and theoretically understand why it would be practical for our intents and purposes to substitute that ice cream with a frozen yoghurt, because you could eat so much more of the latter and still experience a similar taste/experience. It will amaze you how few people actually practice this tactic consistently, however.

Quickly asking Google to look up vanilla ice cream calories results in the following answer: 207.5 calories per 100 g. What does a vanilla froyo measure up to? Answers range anywhere from 100 to 140 calories per 100 g. The exact number is really not important, just think about the difference. I understand that different brands have different flavors, and that normal vanilla ice cream might be preferred. However, the "sacrifice" is worth it. The stimulation from the froyo will be very similar to that of the ice cream. Most people use ice cream as a dessert and want to experience a bit of sweetness after a savory meal. The froyo will be close enough to that experience, and you better believe this. Maybe it won't feel like it the very first time, but it will eventually. You can even talk yourself into believing that the froyo tastes much better!

Remember that your paradigm guides your thoughts. You choose what you believe. If you talk yourself into believing that you want froyo instead of ice cream, or fried turkey instead of fried bacon, or low-fat popcorn instead of regular potato chips, you eventually will. You'll crave what you eat, and if you replace some of your favorite food choices with 'close enough' alternatives, you'll be amazed at how much you can enjoy your life while still making progress.

The art of replacing is one of the most underutilized, most potent tactics there is. Do be creative with it and practice it as much as you can. Eventually you'll be much fuller, more often than before, while still enjoying the same type of lifestyle as you used to.

Naturally, replacement and intermittent fasting can be used simultaneously. In fact, combining them is an act of creativity. Whenever you start coming up with your own ideas, you're demonstrating that you're becoming conscious about your food decisions. I want to emphasize this as it's a sign that you're making progress. It's an important stage and it deserves some reflection.

Try to think of the most important food-related or health-related principle you've learned and practiced. The principle of choice may be different from person to person and, usually, the most important principle turns out to be the one that's been most helpful to the individual. Some people are never the same after they've learned that feelings of hunger can be reinterpreted as a 'minor inconvenience' rather than a 'you-need-to-eat alarm.' Others may swear that eating fixed units of food makes life and transforming simpler than ever before.

The first time on a journey of my own, the most enlightening aspect was the true caloric cost of food choices. A salad with sprinkled nuts on top and a piece of bread on the side suddenly became off limits once I realized this was just as calorically dense as a pizza and didn't even fill me up. I realized that just because nuts contain healthy fats and that a salad is commonly thought of as the 'light option,' it doesn't mean unmeasured quantities can go into my diet.

As soon as it dawned on me that I had the means to reduce starvation to a minimum and still transform my appearance, something happened. My mental paradigm shifted drastically. Most of what I knew about food had been conventional wisdom, which was, and still is, embarrassing to admit. As soon as the mental shift happened, pragmatic decisions guided my behavior. Breakfast was no longer a necessity. A bowl of broccoli with nothing else could be lunch, dinner, or a snack, depending on where I was and what I had to do. Some days, food wasn't necessary at all. At other times, one meal and ten beers were the way to go. As long as the choices were in alignment with my goals, they were good choices.

To me, pragmatic choices had the greatest impact. To you, it may be intermittent fasting or something else. Consider what principle or concept helps you the most and strive to always rely on it. If you have the fundamentals down, results will come eventually. You won't easily be able to escape the fact that you need to be aware of your calories and weight, but you'll be able to keep track of and understand your digits better if you know how to routinely behave on a daily basis. If you do intermittent fasting, you only need to calculate your calories one to three times per day. If you eat in units, calculating calories is as easy as adding two plus two. If you understand yourself and what works best for you, you can design a lifestyle that's simple and enjoyable, which also takes you towards your goal.

Macronutrients and Consequences

It's fair to say that this book is repetitive, but I think this is necessary. New knowledge sometimes takes a while to assimilate. However, if we keep exposing ourselves to ideas, new and old, we're making important steps towards progress and learning. Now, as you consistently gather experience about how you emotionally react to hunger, collect factual data about how you're eating, and practice the skill of controlling what you eat on a daily basis, you're exposing yourself to everything that's necessary to learn the skill of transforming.

You really do have most of the body transforming knowledge you need to last you a lifetime. Please keep this in mind as we talk about macronutrients. It's good to be familiar with what they are, but you honestly don't need this knowledge as long as you have common sense. What this means will be elaborated on when the subject of alcohol is put into the mix. Anyway, here goes.

I chose to omit 'macros' at the beginning of the book. Too much information can easily become the opposite of simple, which is the first priority of this book. This far in, it's safer to introduce them. So, to put it simply, macronutrients is a collective term for carbohydrates, proteins, and fats. Basically, our food is made out of those three components. Why you've probably come across people who talk about tracking macros and fitting their meals into their macros is because of the idea that our bodies demand certain ratios of each category (the categories being fats, carbs, and proteins, of course).

This is of course valid; we do need to feed our bodies with the right types of fuels in the right amounts. However, my perspective on the matter of worrying about macronutrients is this: a quick gut check will do the same trick for most people on this planet. Just think about how you're feeling on different foods and adjust your diet in accordance with what you want to achieve.

Optimizing your macros is necessary if you're a professional athlete, but most normal people only need to make a few conscious food choices to achieve all the results they need. If the latter person more closely resembles you, you can save an immense amount of time and energy if you ignore macros and focus on using common sense instead. I'll try to illustrate this reasoning in practice with a little help from alcohol.

When I was a few years younger and studied, life was pretty much only about studying, working, working out, and having an enjoyable time. This usually involved alcohol and friends. Everyone is different and has different perspectives on what equals fun recreation, but most everyone agrees that having an enjoyable time is an indispensable necessity of life. In case you're similarly inclined to me, a few drinks with good friends are moments you don't want to pass up on. What helped me get two goods at the same time, a body transformation *and* good times with friends, was an understanding of the costs and sacrifices, as well as a willingness to accept them.

What am I talking about, more exactly? Well, if I knew my friends had planned to meet up in the city on Friday evening, I wasn't going to miss it. That meant I would exercise as usual that Friday, skip eating, and instead save room for ten pints of beer during the evening. We could spend time just as we always had, and it was great! Can you imagine how I felt the next day, however? Actually, not that awful, but pretty awful. When you know what you're getting yourself into, you're prepared to deal with the downside. Waking up after ten beers and no food could cause a bit of a headache. Lots of water, several cups of coffee, and about 400 g. of turkey (360 calories in my case) usually cured me. I could then repeat the process on the Saturday, with a workout, and another amazing night with friends, and I usually did.

This was far from the healthiest thing in the world, but that wasn't the point. The purpose was to have a nice body, and to enjoy myself with friends. I didn't need macronutrients to understand the consequences of my choices. Just to point out something, however: is two nights out less healthy than years of overeating and no exercise? It's something to think about. I'm not a pedigree of humanity; all I can say is that you don't have to be one just to have a nice-looking and healthy body. Luckily, you can still be a good person, regardless of unhealthy habits, and that's a lot better than the reverse. The good eventually outweighs the bad if we practice consistency and patience in other areas.

Although the above anecdote related to alcohol, it naturally applies to other guilty pleasures too. The core issue that you need to resolve is whether you understand the consequences of your actions, and if you're willing to accept them. Be mindful, just as you are with your food. With thought and conscious effort, you can have what you envision, be it the nice body, the fun, the longevity, or all of it.

Preparation for Next Week

For next week, you'll receive a bit more of a challenge than previously. The reason for this is that you need to realize how competent you've become over the last few weeks. Remember, you'll only be tasked with objectives you have the means to conquer. So, for next week, you'll reduce your calories by 200. Just prepare to take on next week a day at a time. You can do this!

Week 7
Diets

Summary of what you'll be doing

- Remaining consistent with your *new* caloric target (200 calories less).

- Tracking your calories on your smartphone on a daily basis.

- Documenting your weight every morning.

- Documenting your total calories every evening.

- Learning about various diets.

- **Optional task:** Your first reset (only available on the last day of the week).

Extra important during this week

- Sticking with your calorie target is absolutely essential—priority number one.

- If you feel it won't compromise your first priority *do* try out different foods from various diets. Exposure to different diets is good for the long term.

An Important Distinction

Tracking calories is *not* a diet. It's a pragmatic means to achieve results. What you choose to do with your calories is what's called your diet. Many fad diets become trendy for a while, then die out. Usually, results from such diets are minimal or short lived. There are a few diets, however, which people have had consistent success with over extended periods of time. This week, you'll be exposed to a few of these.

Understanding what types of diets suit you well will be immensely beneficial in the long term, so I urge you to play around with food choices this week. One very important caveat, however; don't compromise your (pretty low) caloric target for this week. It's better that you skip experimenting than miss your calorie target, just to be clear.

Diets and Calorie Tracking

The distinction I just mentioned is really important. Diet, tracking calories, and strategies for hunger control all are separate matters. In this book, we approach all topics from a perspective of wanting to achieve results using some of the simplest, most sustainable methods that have already worked for other people. If lasting results are what matters in the end, my perspective is that your choice of diet and strategies for hunger control should always agree with your personal preferences and inclinations. However, in the matters of tracking calories, there's little room for personalization. I'm about to explain what I mean by making a few pretty sweeping statements. Please bear with me, however, as I try to explain my reasoning.

Calories matter to all humans, it's undeniable and indisputable. On a personal note, my opinion is that individuals who want to transform should start by getting an accurate understanding of their caloric needs and then proceed to acquire the ability to control their caloric intake (which is what we're doing). It's simply the most pragmatic way of securing results because nothing is left to chance.

By monitoring calories and weight, results become *tangible* and *adjustable*. With data about yourself, and an understanding of it, you can always manipulate the caloric input towards a desired physique, be it a leaner or a bigger one. My opinion is that once an understanding of your caloric needs is truly mastered and innate, you can then proceed to consider other methods than calorie counting if you want to (although I'm hesitant to recommend it).

Although many people have different ideas on how results are best achieved, I think there's at least consensus around the idea that *understanding* calories is mandatory, regardless of whether everyone is a proponent of tracking them or not. Why I would hesitate to recommend anyone to stop tracking calories is this (as I've already stated before): the act of tracking gives you *certainty* and *confidence*, and it eventually becomes so simple to do that you have to spend less than five minutes a day on it! That's why I'm, admittedly quite stubbornly, of the opinion that there's no better way to achieve results than to be mindful about food choices and by tracking your essential numbers (calories and weight).

Whenever a diet alone is said to produce transformative results, I raise a cautioning finger mentally. It's not that certain diets aren't helpful or contribute to the results but, fundamentally, it's the individual's consistent and correct *behavior* that causes the change. I can't overstate how important this point is. You, dear reader, are the commander in chief of your body; never be mistaken about this.

So, with the above (quite lengthy, but very important) rambling in mind, diet is always up to you, but there's no budging on the calorie tracking part.

Finally, when it comes to hunger control, many seem to achieve success with eating windows, aka intermittent fasting, as I've already mentioned. Experimenting with eating windows and diet is, by far, the best way I've found to resolve my own struggles with hunger. Even if you don't want to try intermittent fasting, I still recommend you experiment throughout your continued journey. The more you find out what works for you, the simpler everything becomes. Hang in there and try to enjoy the process for what it is!

Simple and Voluminous Foods

This diet is one of my own making. It's ridiculously simple and I've relied heavily on it during my own transformation journeys. The essential idea is consuming simple, voluminous foods—that's it. *Simple*, as in easy to prepare, easy to take with you, or easy to find when on the run. *Voluminous*, as in relatively low calorie content for a generous portion of food.

Just to give a quick example, what's a type of food that's both simple and voluminous? Broccoli. This would thus be part of a simple, voluminous diet, either as a full meal or as a significant portion of a meal. Sounds tremendously boring, right? The thing I've found after more than a decade, however, is that it's more fun overall to not go hungry all the time, rather than eating something very tasty that doesn't fill me up as much. Voluminous foods will fill you up the most and you'll learn to love them for it. That the food also is simple, in the sense just mentioned, means it's less likely one messes up due to stress. If a great filling meal is always just five minutes away, you'll never have to make rash food decisions that potentially mess up the calorie target for the day.

This type of diet, or perhaps principle of eating, isn't just based on my own experience, but also on a lot of wise people's suggestions. If you want your results to last, you eventually find ways to make it easier for yourself. What's *simple* will, of course, vary from person to person, and the most important thing is that the food choices you make are adjusted to your personal needs and circumstances. In my own case, stress and duties fill up most of my days. I wouldn't have the time to prepare macronutrient-optimal meals that taste like heaven and couldn't overcome the struggle to justify the amount of money it would cost me to outsource every meal for an extended period. It's not that there aren't a lot of great recipes for good-tasting, healthy food out there. These recipes just aren't always as practical or applicable to everyday life as I would need them to be.

When normal days are stuffed with musts and stress, I've chosen to replace high food variance, great taste, and macronutrient optimization with foods that have high practicality, low price, and relatively low calorie content (they're voluminous). This doesn't mean I'm a proponent of bad-tasting, unhealthy food. It means I just want to be as full as possible, at the lowest possible cost, without sacrificing my health. It's a form of 'satisficing' or choosing the pragmatic rather than the ideal option (see economist Herbert Simon's work for more info). This usually means that I consume a lot of oatmeal, ham, baked potatoes, and cabbage, for example. Here's a brief list of foods that are both practical and voluminous, so do what you want with them!

- Cabbage
- Ham
- Turkey
- Rice cakes
- Egg whites
- Broccoli
- Watermelon
- Diet ice cream (with stewed raspberries)

Bro Foods

In case you've never got what a 'bro' is, go watch Dom Mazzetti's YouTube channel, 'brosciencelife'. He portrays and satirizes the ultimate bro, and it's very entertaining. Basically, a bro is your stereotypical self-proclaimed 'alpha male' who loves everything about the gym.

Regardless of what anyone says about bros, there's a lot of wisdom in them, so don't underestimate them. Bros are stereotypically known for applying pseudoscience to both diet and exercise, but that's actually only a half-truth. Bros share details about what they've done to achieve their physique. It's a genre more resembling memoir than empirical science, and the receiver of the information should thus utilize it as such—as personal reflections on an individual's journey, which may or may not be suitable for another individual with different genetics or goals, rather than as an endeavor to find facts and truths.

The stereotypical bro would eat something like chicken and rice, or tilapia and asparagus, seven times a day, consuming various blends of vitamins and shakes, etc. This is, of course, an exaggeration, but hopefully the point gets across. The bro tends to stick to a diet where the meal frequency is high, the protein consumption is high, and where clean versus dirty foods are a thing.

It's up to you to decipher whether the information a bro shares would work for you, but all I can tell you is this: some of the bros really, and I mean *really* know what they're doing with their own bodies. Just be careful about who you listen to; you really need to be critical about the information and its applicability to you.

Wholefoods, Plant-Based Diet

Now this diet is really special. There's an entire book about it called *The China Study*, which is a highly controversial book about the wholefoods, plant-based diet and its health benefits. I do recommend you read it at some point because it provokes a lot of thought. Now, I'm not able to confirm or dismiss the information in the book, but I can at least tell you that I appreciate many of the fundamental points that it makes. Whole, plant-based foods are both healthy and generally underutilized by modern consumers, and it's pretty safe to say most of us would benefit from, and feel a hell of a lot better with, more plant-based wholefoods in our diets. Whether or not this is *the* diet of all diets is just not for me to say.

The only thing I can say without stepping out of bounds is that if you're eating like me, you'll benefit from applying the ideas from the wholefoods, plant-based diet, because there's too little of this type of food in the regular diet. Whether you want to apply everything that the book proposes or not is up to you. You'll not become worse off from reading the book and making your mind up about the contents yourself. So, if you're interested in this type of diet and lifestyle, read *The China Study*. If you're satisfied with your current diet, save the read for later, when you need new motivation.

Implementing a New Diet

Trying a new diet may feel exciting and fun for a few days, or even a full week or two. Just remember, however, that diets in themselves aren't magical. There will be no drastic increases or decreases in your metabolism, even though you may 'feel something' within your body during this time. A change of diet may affect how your stomach feels, or your mood in general. If the change feels positive, that's all good, but you shouldn't misconstrue these short-term contrasts for improvements or faster results. Perhaps a lesser amount of carbs makes you less sleepy after eating. Perhaps you feel more energized from eating more carbs than before. These effects are all fine and good, but they won't make a drastic difference to your progress, and I can't repeat this too many times.

Your progress will keep coming at the same speed it usually does, even though you may feel slightly different. What a diet can do well, and what you should look for, is one that keeps you full and makes you feel energized during the right hours of the day (that is, during work, and potentially also during workouts). That's it. If you feel full and have energy, while being able to stick with your calorie target, you've got it.

Please note, however, that 'full' is a relative term. You'll feel less and less full the longer you get into the transformation process— that's how it's supposed to be. So, don't switch diets frequently in hopes of finding something that makes you feel full all the time, because you likely won't. If you struggle with hunger, I suggest you try the simple, voluminous foods combined with intermittent fasting. It takes a week or two to get used to, but then it usually does wonders for the task of controlling hunger.

Your Optional Task This Week

At this stage, you have the opportunity to make a choice. Please note that this option only exists on the last day of week 7. If everything is going smoothly and you're enjoying the process, I suggest you discard the possibility of your first reset for now and use it at a time when you need it more. However, if you're struggling with hunger right now, stay with me!

It's time to do a quick reboot of your system. All it really is, is an extra-large meal, but it may have a significant effect on you. If you've been particularly hungry the last few days, this is what you've been waiting for. It's one day where you get to feel the sensation of being completely full again.

Don't take this day as an invitation for you to pig out on anything you would like, because that's not what's supposed to happen. Rather, on this one day, you get to eat a few extra portions of dinner until you're completely full. In practice, this means that you go about your day as you normally would, but that (normal) dinner is extra-large. The point is that you get to feel completely full for one day and get a chance to reset your mental and physical systems a bit. Usually, this type of activity leads to extra energy and high spirits for many days to come.

A small reset is supposed to reduce the risk of 'fuck it' moments. If you never get to feel full, your mind may start playing games, which can lead to binge eating and anxiety. If, on the other hand, there are moments when you get to reset your hunger, you may have an easier time adhering to calorie targets in the long run.

Please keep in mind that we're talking about one day, and it's truly supposed to be only one. These resets are meant to be used very sparingly. Only a few weeks after having a reset is when you should start thinking about another reset. Just be cautious and don't overuse them. They're supposed to reset you, not simply comfort you. Pay attention to when you really need a reset, and when you're just hungry. The former situation is when you think about a reset; during the latter one you never do.

Preparation for Next Week

For next week, we won't make any changes to your calories. This, again, means that your preparation is mental. As always, it's essential that you remain with the caloric target.

By this time, you may have started to notice a bit of resistance in terms of hunger, fatigue, doubting whether you're getting results or not, etc. Don't worry, however; these feelings and thoughts are both natural and normal. It's now of the highest importance that you remain patient. You *are* getting there, and you need to keep reminding yourself about this in the coming week.

There are a lot of things that can brighten your day, which aren't food related, and we'll talk about this during next week. Stay strong!

Week 8
Rewarding Yourself While Keeping Momentum

Summary of what you'll be doing

- Remaining consistent with your caloric target (same as last week).

- Tracking your calories on your smartphone on a daily basis.

- Documenting your weight every morning.

- Documenting your total calories every evening.

- **Task:** Reward yourself.

Extra important during this week

- Make sure you give yourself enough props for making it this far. It doesn't matter if you're not at your ideal body yet, because it's only a matter of time until you're there. *Enjoy the journey*.

Momentum

The discussion about resets in the previous week was filled with cautionary words, and there's a reason for this. A succession of good days—that is, days of adherence to your calorie target—takes energy and time to work up to. Once you've got up to speed, however, you have momentum, and ensuing good days are easier to achieve.

Now, what tends to happen when stepping out of the normal routine, when acting against the momentum that's been built up—it could be a reset or simply a day where all calories come from new places (drinks or candy, for instance)—is that you very quickly lose all the momentum, and coming days become more of a struggle than they've been during recent weeks.

Choosing to have days 'off routine' can be a risky business if you aren't prepared for the potential loss of momentum. If you're prepared for an eventual period of extra resistance, you can do whatever you want. What you must clarify to yourself is whether any special meal or drink is worth the extra resistance. If you struggle with consistency, I recommend you consume as few off-routine calories as possible, because such calories may complicate things unnecessarily. If things are running smoothly, as I said before, you can do whatever you want, as long as you're within the calorie target.

Please note that momentum doesn't necessarily have to end with an off-routine day, but there's risk of added resistance involved in such choices. This is the primary reason I'm hesitant to recommend ad lib diets. It's not that they don't work, it's just that most people struggle more with adherence and consistency with such diets that other ones. Routine and an increasing momentum, gained from simple and uniform diets such as simple and voluminous, and low carb, for instance, simplify the practice of the principle of consistency. Ad lib diets generate just as much progress, but that progress may be tougher to sustain due to the lack of momentum.

Everyone is different, and for some momentum may very well be just as present in an ad lib diet as in a more uniform one. Just think about this, however: most people's lack of results is due to a lack of consistency. It's not the diet that's the issue, you just want consistency. So, if there's any way you can increase consistency and adherence, you want to go there. Risking progress for a more 'free and tasty' diet won't be worth it for most. Consistency and patience get you your results, and that's the only thing that matters in the end. Build momentum, keep at it, and stay strong! Few ever get further than two weeks into a transformation, so if you've got this far, you can be proud of yourself. Just keep at it and try to have as much fun as you can, because you're getting there!

Your Task This Week

Leading up to this week, I mentioned that there are ways to brighten your day that aren't food related. This is what it's now time for. This far into the game, you should start noticing a few changes in your body. There are a few ways to make the changes stand out. First, you can take a few more pictures. Compare today's pictures with the pictures you took on day one, and pay attention to the details of your stomach, arms, shoulders, legs, and face. In case you think the mirror looks the same all the time (which we've already talked about), the pictures can reveal what the mirror can't, and it's usually quite impressive to see what's been going on over the last few weeks.

Another way to notice changes is in the clothes you wear. If you have a favorite item that you've used many, many times, that same item may have a different fit suddenly. Pay attention to how your clothes used to fit, and how they fit now. Are they looser than usual? Do you somehow look a bit different, even though you wear the same clothes as usual? How your clothes fit and look on you reveals a lot about your body, and it's one of the best ways to measure your progress.

Now, if you've actually noticed positive changes—and this is regardless of whether the changes are huge or minor, if they're as big as you anticipated, or if no one but you notices—you deserve a reward. You deserve to feel good about yourself, and you deserve to treat yourself to something special. Of course, I'm not talking about a big meal that potentially interrupts momentum or leads to future anxiety; I'm talking about a vanity reward. If you've made progress, buy a nice piece of clothing for yourself, preferably one that accentuates your results.

Are your legs slimmer than before? Do your arms look better than ever? Set aside something like $50–$100 (or an equivalent) for a nice new outfit. This might include a high-quality shirt that reveals your figure, a nice pair of jeans that have a slimmer fit, or similar. Dare to show off your progress (especially to yourself)—you really deserve it. Be confident and proud about the fact you've accomplished something immensely important. Other people will notice your results if you notice them first, so be honest with yourself. Have you made progress? Give yourself a pat on the back, and wear something that articulates your progress.

It's important for you to remember that the results you've thus far gotten are not the end-all or be-all. This is your first step on a long journey, and there's no telling where you might end up if you stay consistent. The dream about the perfect body is vividly real if you approach that goal with knowledge and control. You've already proved that you're able to control your body by tracking calories, weight, and achieving results. Stay on the path and realize that whatever progress you've so far achieved is only part of the results you'll achieve during years to come.

If results are achievable in a matter of a few weeks, imagine what one or two years of progress would look like. The process gets easier the more you do it, and soon enough results will come almost automatically, because your autopilot is set on results and wellbeing, both physical and mental. Great job so far! Stay strong!

Exceptions

Although I've talked a lot about effort and consistency, there are still a few more related things to be said about the subjects. In the real world, where 'life' takes place, we'll eventually stumble upon various 'disruptions.' Call them what you want, but these are the social events or important work-related duties that come up at times, and which you can't easily ignore (or shouldn't ignore).

Why they're called 'disruptions' is simply because they and similar events may disrupt our preferred daily routine and momentum. At times when we're facing a disrupting event, when sub-optimal food choices are likely to be necessary, it's very easy to disregard the entire day, and internally promise to 'get back in order tomorrow.' However, it's precisely this tendency we want to avoid. Even if you have dinner and a glass of wine with an important customer at work, or eat cake at a kid's birthday party, it's still possible to take a long walk and exercise for fifteen minutes (even if you're wearing a suit during the walk and exercise in the bathroom before showering). Even if your effort is minuscule compared to what you're normally able to do, it's immensely important you still do it.

One doughnut will *not* ruin anything. One doughnut is *not* an invitation to pig out. A late dinner with wine does *not* hinder anyone from taking a forty-minute walk before bed. Dinner can still be cabbage and turkey, even if you messed up your first meal due to a work-related errand requiring you to have a fat burger. The essential principle is that you let exceptions be exceptions.

Don't let anything get in the way of your 'enough' (your daily walk/tracking of calories/daily exercise, etc.), because it just isn't necessary. It's not always easy to do what you consider enough, especially when opposing duties require your time and energy, but that's mostly because our minds play tricks with us. We get used to doing things in a certain way, and at times we forget that we're free to make our own rules. Who says raw cabbage isn't breakfast food? Why shouldn't you work out at 3 a.m. in the morning? A walk is a walk is a walk, and a good decision is too, regardless of how many sub-optimal ones were made previously.

Always strive to make good decisions, and don't feel bad or like giving up just because you made one or a few sub-optimal ones. Perhaps you might even call the latter ones *necessary* decisions. The point is that as long as you always strive to make good decisions, the occasional sub-optimal ones become true exceptions, and true exceptions will always be completely fine.

Preparation for Next Week

Soon enough, your ten-week journey will be finished and we'll enter into the third part of this book, which is about your continued journey and longevity. At that point, there's a period of reflection and a larger reset of the system, but more on that later. Before the current part of your journey is completed, there are just over two weeks to go. During these two weeks, a few details are to get extra attention.

At this stage, the calorie target is as important as always. For next week, you're to reduce your calories by another 200. Although you should just hit your target as usual, I understand and appreciate that this might feel a bit more difficult this time around. Many of you may be a bit fed up with being hungry all the time, especially this far into the process. What I'm urging you to do at this point is to mentally prepare to 'stick it out' a bit harder than usual during the last two weeks, because you may need it.

Something to keep in mind when things get rough is that you soon enter a period where you reset the system. During the reset you'll erase the hunger and forget you even experienced it—trust me. Be extra stubborn with the calorie target during these last two weeks. You may experience a bit of extra resistance—best-case scenario, you won't, but most do. You need to remind yourself that this resistance is something very temporary, and that it won't affect you more than as momentary hunger, which you already know you can handle.

Something else that's essential during the last two weeks is clever use of hunger tactics. If you start feeling very hungry, I recommend you think of using a potent old trick of mine: take a walk to a nearby store, buy a nice, low-calorie treat (like a watermelon), and walk back home. The walk should be at least thirty minutes there and back. If you're still hungry after the walk, you can consider eating the treat. Not only is this trick a peaceful and potent distraction from hunger, but you'll also be able to focus on your thoughts and/or the audio you're listening to. Do have this strategy in mind during the last two weeks.

As I've already pointed out, you have 200 fewer calories to play with. You'll also be tasked with doing cardio for the sake of assisting your weight loss. This is a new introduction as compared to the other weeks. I can't overstate how important it is that you brace yourself for the coming week. If you're mentally prepared, you'll conquer the next week with a smile. You just need to be prepared for your body's attempts to trick you into believing that you need to overeat.

Week 9
Initiating the Spurt

Summary of what you'll be doing

- Remaining consistent with your *new* caloric target (200 calories less).

- Tracking your calories on your smartphone on a daily basis.

- Documenting your weight every morning.

- Documenting your total calories every evening.

- **Task:** Take two to four walks during this week.

Extra important during this week

- This is a tougher week than the previous ones. Not only are you on an all-time caloric low, but cardio is to be added. Remaining positive and being mentally strong is absolutely essential this week. You *will* get through it.

Your Task This Week

Although you might come across additional emotional resistance this week, cardio is still going to be included as a task. You should get the hint that this is important, as it's the first thing I cover during this week. There's no reason to fear this inclusion, however, as this task isn't intended to feel like hard work. Not at all. Although we name this task/activity cardio, we're simply talking about taking a long walk.

The idea is that you add between two and four *additional* walks of forty minutes (not more, not less) during this week. This means that if you already take walks regularly, you'll add these two to four walks on top of what you already do.

During the last two weeks of your journey, we're adding these walks to try to increase the caloric deficit you're already on, but without removing additional calories. Although we've previously discussed how you can't outwork too many calories, and how excessive activity won't lead to more results, it's still important to have a bit more of a nuanced understanding of activity and cardio.

There *is* a time and a place for activity and cardio. As we proceed to the last two weeks of this part of your journey, you've put in the prerequisite work to get a little additional benefit from just that. With several weeks of getting your body used to low calories, spicing up your routine with a little bit of additional cardio often works as a catalyst for that last piece of weight that's a bit more stubborn to lose. Imagine what your new, lower calorie target combined with a little extra cardio might do for you. Try to enjoy it!

Things to Listen to During Cardio

A cardio session can be anything from running, to swimming, to long walks, and by now it's probably very clear that I prefer long walks. The low intensity makes the activity pleasurable. To enhance the experience and avoid it becoming dull, I recommend headphones and audio. Getting away from everything for thirty to sixty minutes every day, and getting to listen to whatever you want, soon becomes a favorite segment of the day for many people. Really try to see that you're taking care of your physical and mental self on these walks and enjoy the feeling of doing good while also feeling good.

Here are a few ideas of things to listen to during your cardio sessions:

- **A complete album, from start to finish.** Don't underestimate this one. An album often brings out a sense of dynamics, which single songs out of order may not be able to reveal. Choose an artiste you really appreciate and listen to one of their classic albums from start to finish. At times, there's nothing better than this.

- **Listen to an informative podcast.** There are many great podcasts out there. My suggestion is that you pick something that's not only entertaining, but that also supplies some sort of informative value for you. The topic is up to you to choose. Some people love discussions about clothes or cars, while others prefer podcasts about cooking or movies. Pick your poison!

- **Audiobooks.** This is a big one. If cardio plus audiobooks becomes habitual, there's immense growth potential to realize. According to various media outlets such as INC.com and FastCompany.com, American CEOs read approximately one book every week of the year. If you walk several days a week, you'll be able to consume close to the same number of books as these CEOs, and isn't that pretty amazing?

The True Cost

What you're experiencing on a day-to-day basis during this week is the true cost of a body transformation. The hunger, the tiredness, the time invested in walking, etc. No matter how much we would be willing to pay for someone or something else to do this work for us, it's still you and I that must pay for ourselves, the currency being the effort of actually doing it. The number of things you've been willing to do right for the past weeks and months are equal to the type of results you've now achieved—nothing more, nothing less. Not even illegal supplements can do the work for you; you would still have to keep track of your food to achieve your desired results.

With your recent efforts fresh in mind, really ponder what the price for a transformation comes to. Having control of your body and complete independence usually adds up to a worthwhile reward. Complete control over your body is a skill that could have cost even more time and effort, and still be worth it.

If we take a step back and view the concept of controlling your body from a larger perspective, it's one of the most worthwhile investments you could ever make in a lifetime. Just think about what the Dalai Lama said when asked what surprised him most about humanity:

Man. Because he sacrifices his health in order to make money. Then he sacrifices money to recuperate his health. And then he is so anxious about the future that he does not enjoy the present; the result being that he does not live in the present or the future; he lives as if he is never going to die, and then dies having never really lived. ***Dalai Lama***

You don't have to be very spiritual to appreciate the underlying truth he's getting at. It's a pattern that's very recognizable, perhaps even close to us. Deteriorating health is a harsh and oftentimes very tragic matter of life, and it's not always possible to do anything about the situation. Don't get stuck in the thought but think about someone you care about who turned sicker and sicker with age. Nothing in this world makes up for our loved ones—no money, drug, or replacement.

Now, just try to imagine that you and your family have the means to reduce the risk for deteriorating health; wouldn't it be worth anything in the world? A sustainable lifestyle where you're able to control and take care of your body is just that risk reducer. The price you pay for a lifetime of immeasurable value is the energy you spend on being mindful about food, and your eventual implementation of exercise and cardio.

The cost of transforming and controlling your body is one thing, but what you receive back is far more important. That you get to choose your appearance is one thing (and it's a fantastic thing), but the more important aspect is the fact that you get to be in control of your own life, and that you get to enjoy your life at your highest potential for more years than you otherwise would. Take care of yourself, really. You'll thank yourself years and decades from now.

Dealing with the Social Aspects

When it comes to the short-term perspective, meaning the ten or so weeks where the focus is on transforming your appearance, one of the absolute toughest aspects to handle is the 'social' one. I'm not talking so much about your social life, although that also can be a bit trickier to navigate. No, I'm referring to the tendency that you receive increasingly frequent remarks about your lifestyle decisions.

When embarking on a journey like the one you're currently on, it becomes increasingly apparent that food is a huge part of our lives. A meal is something we share with people we care about. Eating is oftentimes the preferred activity when we plan a night of fun with our friends. Since you're not eating purely for pleasure, but more so with an intention to fuel your body and feel well (especially during these last two weeks of the transformation), a large part of your social life will be affected. If you don't have food in common with your friends and family, what do you do to enjoy each other's company? I don't have any good answers because it takes two to tango.

What can be said, however, is that if having an enjoyable time has involved good food for several years, it's a good idea to expect a bit of social resistance. You may be called boring, called out for not being yourself, or for being shallow, etc. Even though you know that what's being said isn't true, you'll feel some pain if you're ever exposed to such feedback from your peer group. We're social creatures and have been for thousands of generations. The mental cues tied to our social standing are so ingrained that whether our social group accepts us or not is a top priority. Pain from social rejection, even if minuscule, is unavoidable.

Although there's little we can do about the pain that comes from our social brains, you can at least prepare for some common situations. If you expect the pain, and you remember that this current situation is temporary, you may just be a little more resilient than you otherwise would have been.

Remarks can come anytime we find ourselves in a social setting, but especially when food is involved (which is a natural occurrence for most people three to five times a day). Be especially ready during lunchtime at work and during social events with friends. The least painful remark comes from the curious acquaintance who asks questions out of interest:

"Have you lost weight?"

"What's your secret?"

"Wow, is that all you get to eat?"

"Aren't you hungry all the time?"

This is usually not an issue. If you have to repeat yourself a dozen times during the same meal, then it can be a bit annoying. If it comes to having to justify your choices, then it becomes truly annoying.

One of the few things that can be worse than having to justify your decisions (when no one else has to justify theirs), is when you come upon outright unsolicited opinions. Even though you wouldn't remark on your acquaintance's fourth lunchtime cheeseburger of the week, and even though they wouldn't remark on yours either, had you had a similar lifestyle, you may nonetheless be the primary receiver of unsolicited opinions, most likely because your food choices consistently conflict with what's considered 'normal' or 'you.'

"I prefer to enjoy my life."

"I heard it's unhealthy to starve like that."

"You should vary your meals more, the body needs variance."

"I'm glad I'm not as shallow. I wouldn't manage eating nothing."

The list could go on, but the point should be clear enough. Be prepared to meet social resistance and be prepared that it most likely will affect you, like it or not. We're social creatures, and the social aspect is one of the harder ones to tackle.

The Scale is Erratic

The scale will start becoming erratic during the transformation journey. At first, you may see quite steady declines in weight, which seems very logical, because it feels like a cause and effect type of equation. However, weight loss is unfortunately not linear, and the further you get into the journey, the stranger things are likely to become.

Even if you do everything right, consume the right number of calories, and even add exercise and some cardio, you may put *on* a few grams/pounds. Not only does this make you wonder whether 'the system' is broken, but it can also feel incredibly unfair. The thing is this: every right decision you make is a step forward, regardless of whether you can see any immediate results. First, the feedback you get from your efforts has a lag time. Second, your results may come in shapes and forms other than just weight loss. Does your face look slimmer? Does the fat on your body 'sit' differently than previously? Are you slightly more vascular in certain places? These can all be indicators of progress, regardless of what the scale tells you.

What you must understand is that good decisions always matter, regardless of whether it's possible to see results or not. The lag time is real, and it mustn't distract you from the things you know you should do—eat according to your target calories and, currently, also do cardio.

Let weight loss be undulating. Keep being consistent yourself and trust your process. The journey isn't really eight or ten weeks, it's a lifetime one, and incremental progress and undulating conditioning (appearance-wise) of your body is part of the journey. Appreciate it and try to enjoy it. If you know you're doing the right thing, you never have to worry. The feedback *will* come, eventually.

Just a few words of caution: don't try to force immediate feedback/results by drastically reducing your calories or increasing your exercise or cardio. Just stick to your targets and be confident. If you can let go of the need for immediate feedback, which may occur in the beginning, but becomes less and less prevalent the more aligned with your body you get, you'll start nurturing a feeling of certainty and confidence.

Getting in control of your body— or 'mastering it' we might even say for the sake of this analogy—is just like achieving mastery in any other activity or field. Going from being a complete newbie to reaching amateur levels of skill or proficiency is a short journey. Advancing to intermediate levels requires time, patience, and resilience. Masters are usually driven by a higher purpose, leading them to invest years and years to achieve incremental progress.

Wanting to become healthy and fit for your family's sake is a higher purpose. Wanting to improve one's body to more easily be able to find the love of one's life is a higher purpose. Wanting to go through a transformation to inspire others to do the same is a higher purpose. The process takes time, but it's worth it. You're not only doing it for yourself, but most likely for others too. You're becoming a master, slowly and steadily. Let the process take the time it needs and try to enjoy the journey as much as possible.

Preparation for Next Week

The final week will be much like this one. We initiated what can best be described as a 'spurt' during the current week (hence the chapter title), meaning that we ramped up all parameters and spent a lot of mental energy giving our very best effort to this transformation for a short period of time. It takes time and effort to work up to a spurt, which you've diligently invested, so don't misconstrue these efforts as an attempt to shortcut the process. The spurt *is* part of the process.

Next week, the spurt is finalized, and it's time for even more effort. We're once more to remove 200 calories, making your target the lowest you'll have it for a good while. The added cardio from this week will remain intact too, meaning that the additional two to four walks are to be done too.

After this last week, you'll have plenty of time to reset your system and plan out how you're to achieve additional results in the future, so don't worry about anything other than completing the spurt during last week.

Week 10
Finalizing the Spurt

Summary of what you'll be doing

- Remaining consistent with your *new* caloric target (200 calories less).

- Tracking your calories on your smartphone on a daily basis.

- Documenting your weight every morning.

- Documenting your total calories every evening.

- **Task:** Take two to four walks during this week (same as last week).

- **Task:** Take the after picture (last day of the week).

Extra important during this week

- There's a chance some of the days during this week completely suck. Do NOT give into your emotions and instincts in such cases! This is temporary, and after this week you'll get to reset your body thoroughly.

When the Going Gets Tough

Since you're in the midst of the final week, when the general theme is spurting, it's time to be pragmatic at the expense of being conventional. What most people feel during the last few weeks is constant hunger and low energy. The mind feels different too, a sort of focus and clarity is present, almost to the degree that you become increasingly cynical by the day.

The low calories over time play tricks with the mind and affect your overall mood and thoughts. Once you get to satisfy your hunger for a few days in a row (which takes place in a controlled fashion after this week), the world's appearance will change into something more fun and adventurous looking. Before we get there, however, there are a few more days of feeling hungry and drained.

Although I wish I could say that there are magical solutions, I just haven't found any yet. When times are tough, there's usually not much you can do to be relieved from your struggles. I've included some practical things in the chapters contained within this week but, honestly, knowing that it's not a permanent state is about as good as it's going to get at this point.

Managing During This Week

On a day-to-day basis, especially during this phase, it's not only your mood and energy that goes up and down, but your appearance may change almost as often too. Part of this is just your own mind playing tricks on you, but there's also a bit of real change affected by how much water you've been drinking throughout the days, and how many carbs you've consumed in recent times, etc. Please don't let these visible changes affect your behavior, however, as they don't matter very much at the end of the day. If the food behavior is consistent, if there's a trend of a certain positive behavior, the positive results will appear in due time—always be patient.

Just like businesses on the stock market, the body's appearance is volatile. Your appearance may change on a daily basis, for better or for worse, even though your food behavior is as consistent as ever. This volatility never goes away. However, you'll start to fluctuate on new levels as time goes on. If you're on a positive/upward trend, you'll fluctuate in better regions, between more favorable appearances. The volatile situation is always intact—the 'problem' some would say—but it's less of an issue if you keep a long-term perspective. It's better to have the flu than full-blown Ebola, for lack of a better comparison.

When it comes to your mood and how you physically and mentally feel throughout the days on your journey, it's important to understand those daily fluctuations too. On many days you'll feel great; however, some days will be more challenging, and that's just a fact. However, being hungry is overfeared, and you need to remind yourself of this.

Of course, it's a real feeling, and the experience is certainly real, but hunger doesn't affect us nearly as much as many people seem to believe. You need to understand that it's very possible to achieve the same work-related and life-related goals on a good day—that is, a day where everything feels perfect—as on a bad day, where your energy and mood is low. Therefore, there's no need to give in to hunger and say "Fuck it."

What to Do About Hunger

Over the years, I've found a few thought patterns and strategies on managing challenging days that seem to work fairly well, not just for myself, but for others too. Not all days will be challenging, but the key is to be prepared for the days that are. This spurt is likely such a time period for you. It's a bit similar to how a recovering alcoholic might be doing fine for most days of the year, but come Christmas, temptation might be more prevalent than usual.

There are several ways to prevent such and similar situations from becoming a problem, however. One way is to isolate the potentially difficult days and plan an activity over them, which makes it impossible to behave in an unwanted manner. By choosing to make the holiday into normal working days, the potential challenge might be avoided altogether. Of course, one could also choose to celebrate in environments where alcohol is not permitted, but this strategy might not be as foolproof. The essential idea is that the potential problems are anticipated, and that the problems are split into manageable portions; that is, a couple of specific days.

In the cases of the people I've had to do with, weekends and the final spurt (if they ever got there) have been the most common challenging days by far. I urge you to think about different ways to manage your challenging days, and to try different strategies. One of the best methods I've found to tackle my challenging days has been to create a set menu of foods that I only eat during weekends. The key for me is that the food is filling but contains few calories. Taste is secondary for me. During weekends I usually eat a few packs of ham, a few boiled eggs, and popcorn. This may strike some people as weird, but it helps me stay on track. Find out what works for you, and don't hesitate to be unorthodox! It doesn't matter what's considered normal, the important part is that you're achieving the results you want. This is especially important during this week.

Here are some additional practical tips to try—I call this the art of distraction. What we aim to do is distract ourselves from hunger, nothing more, nothing less. If one of these tactics works for you, consider it a tool in your toolbox that you can use from time to time. The fewer times you fall for your hunger emotions and eat something you've not planned to eat, the better it is for you. Clever use of distraction may end up saving you on more than one occasion. Try these things out, and don't hesitate to use some of your own invented methods:

- Have a cup of black coffee.

- This has already been mentioned, but it's worth repeating: take a fifteen-plus-minute walk to a food store. Buy half a watermelon. Walk the fifteen-plus minutes back. If still hungry, consider eating the watermelon.

- Vow to not eat anything until you've watched, listened to, or consumed at least thirty minutes of something you find entertaining—for example, a series, music, a book. You can drink all the water/black coffee/zero-calorie drinks you want in the meantime.

- Sometimes, when nothing else helps, there's a drastic means of distraction that can be used (with extreme caution)—stress at work. Being 100 percent focused on work helps many people forget that they're hungry. Stress has its side effects though, so remember, only use this strategy with caution, and don't learn to rely on it too much.

Remediating Mental and Physical Dips

This process affects both your emotions and physical body, and there will be moments when you feel quite lousy. Having dips and feeling lousy for a few hours is part of the process, and you need to accept it. However, if you constantly feel like fainting, that's not good at all, so drink lots of water, eat something healthy, go take a nap, and then consult a doctor if you haven't improved. A few lousy feelings here and there happen to everyone, though, and they need to be accepted.

Things just get rough at times and there's nothing anyone can do about it. However, there are books treating subjects such as depression, anxiety, and grief (subjects that resemble rough spots during the transformation process, but perhaps to the power of *x*), depending on what you're experiencing. Whenever I've delved into any of the mentioned subjects, there's one golden piece of remedy that always seems to make itself prevalent: focusing on your work and on helping other people.

I couldn't and won't try to prove the potency of this remedy objectively. Instead, I'll refer you to Dale Carnegie's book *How to Stop Worrying and Start Living* and offer a personal anecdote. You can then make up your own mind.

At times, we just want to feel frustrated or tired for a while, and that's completely fine. However, even during seriously dark times, there *is* a way to get relief from our burdens and challenges. By trying to contribute with *something* positive (no matter how small or seemingly insignificant), either to the world in general or to *someone,* we step outside of our own world for a short while to try to improve someone else's reality. Unconditional giving, to the best of one's ability, is about as substantive as the human condition can ever be. Therefore, I urge you think about how you can use your energy to help someone else out, especially if you're feeling down. It doesn't have to be more complicated than giving a stranger a smile or a helping hand or making an unexpected phone call to someone who is lonely.

At the times when the worst blows of my own life occurred (loss, for instance), I also found solace in being consumed by duties. Work and studies were just as tedious as they usually were, but it was impossible to solve tricky problems and deal with personal problems at the same time. I spent the mental energy on duties instead of horrific thoughts. After work, exercising required mental and physical resources yet again. You try focusing on anything other than the fully loaded bar that's in your hands or on your back; it's impossible (if you're able to, you need to increase the weight). Then, at night, there's usually only time to eat food before exhaustion leads to bed.

If the struggle is real for you, focusing (until exhaustion) on duties and trying to be productive is a very potent distraction and remedy. Although you might not be happy at this moment in time, you can still reach a sense of fulfillment and satisfaction for doing the best you can. I don't think constant happiness is the goal of life. Neither is constant productivity and self-sacrifice. The idea of a golden mean makes more sense than both those extremes. Soon enough, there's a wave of happiness for you to ride. Until then, try to enjoy this experience for what it is.

Your Task This Week

By the time you get to this task, it should be the final day of week 10. Before I go on to congratulate you on your tremendous effort, it's time for the last task of this part of the journey: it's time to take an after picture (or pictures, really). This is the happy half of the classic side-by-side transformation photo you can find everywhere online.

You're simply to take the after pictures and put them next to your before pictures. Remember to use something that dates the pictures and to take them in the same place you took your before pictures. Naturally, you can also take pictures in many other places to experiment too! Taking these photos can sometimes be one of the more satisfying rewards, because they're a very tangible type of positive feedback. Enjoy experimenting with lighting and angles and see what your new body looks like!

In Preparation for Part 3

We're now about to enter a different phase of your transformation journey—the reset period. There are a few things we need to know before this, however.

Obviously, for the people who have gone through a transformation, the after pictures are more than just 'normal' pictures. They don't just show the progress that's been made, they have deep internal effects too. Once you realize what you've accomplished, feel the pride and start receiving praise and compliments from friends and strangers, then a longing to hold on to the results starts becoming more and more prevalent.

This effect is positive in the sense that it keeps many from wanting to pig out when they're on their reset period. A word of caution, however. Not wanting to lose results, or immediately wanting more results, tends to lead to a sort of mania for many people, and the idea of being patient is quickly forgotten. This is where you truly need to stop yourself if you're playing around with ideas such as going on a crash diet for supposed additional results, which wouldn't appear, or wouldn't last if they somehow did appear. Remember: *patience*.

The intention of the reset period is to *reset* your mind and body. It seems and sounds so obvious, but sometimes it isn't the most intuitive process when it comes to having to practice it in reality. After being strict for months in a row, looking great, and finally not having to be hungry 80 percent of the time, it may feel perfectly fine to just say 'fuck it' and do whatever one pleases. However, this is precisely the thing we don't want to happen. Breaking momentum and reversing the good habits we've been struggling to build up is the worst possible thing we could do after a transformation journey like the one we've just been on.

Instead, here's what's supposed to happen: for one to three weeks, you'll count your calories and weigh yourself every day, just as usual. However, it's perfectly fine to have an extra portion of food to satisfy your hunger, whether this is when you eat your ordinary lunch, or during dinner, or both. I'm not trying to say you should aim to overeat, just that it's perfectly fine to eat yourself full.

After a day or two of eating a bit more than you've gotten used to during the last few months, you probably won't even need to eat more than you would on an ordinary day. Still, keep tracking calories and weight during your reset weeks. Also strive to do cardio (preferably, walks) two to six times a week (in total, not in addition to what you would normally do).

Do the above, and the following guideline is *decent* enough to follow (I chose the word *decent* because we don't need to be as strict during the reset; it's important that you feel free during it, and that the guideline is 'good enough'—satisficing, again). Imagine that you have 2,000–3,000 extra calories to play around with during each week. If you spend them all on a night out with family or friends or spend 285–430 extra calories a day on food, that's all good and up to you. We'll get more into this in Part 3.

Finally, before proceeding to Part 3, I just wanted to mention that it's more similar to Part 2 than Part 1 in the sense that it contains many entries that function on their own, separately. Although there's a pretty logical chronological order to them (they were conceived as I conducted my little 'field research' for this book, and appear in this book based on the order they were created), they're still individual ideas and thoughts that can be reflected about (and practiced) one at a time for one or a few full days. Just try to take your time with the ideas and keep revisiting the chapters in this book.

I'll be seeing you in Part 3. Until then, enjoy your after pictures!

Part 3

THE CONTINUED JOURNEY

Reset Weeks 1–3
Freedom and Responsibility

What you'll be doing daily

- Counting calories.

- Documenting total calories and weight.

What you'll be doing weekly

- Cardio 2–6 times per week (in total).

Your caloric target for the coming weeks

- Add an extra 2,000–3,000 calories per week (as compared to your last target)—spend as you please.

Congratulations!

Huge congratulations! You've done something for yourself that's immense. I want to stress that you'll feel a lot better during the coming days, and that's because you'll reintroduce more calories to your starving body. Now, I want to make this clear: we're not supposed to pig out right now.

Although you might be in great shape right now, this is an extremely critical time, and we simply must avoid the biggest mistake that it's possible to make in this position: learning a destructive habit. I'm talking about eating disorders and negative food-related behaviors. What we absolutely want to avoid is the tendency to reward ourselves with all the treats we can get our hands on 'because we're worth it' or something similar. It's not that your efforts should go uncelebrated, it's just that we want to celebrate with other things than food.

What happens when you get into great shape and then reward yourself with all your favorite food in the world, which you've craved for almost a month—and I know this from personal experience, because I messed up on this myself and it took about eighteen months to reverse my new destructive habits—is that you experience an incredible high. The comfort of your favorite food combined with your deserved self-worth and sense of accomplishment create a feeling like few other things in the world. The issue here is that this feeling took months of hard work to achieve. It's not the food that makes you feel this great, it's your months-long accomplishment combined with your body's grateful response to calories beyond starvation limits.

I'm not trying to say that you shouldn't have a tasty meal (as in *one* tasty meal) every now and then. If you're not as restricted by calories as you are during an actual transformation period, the tasty meals should definitively be there! What's life if we can't enjoy the pleasures that are available?

No, I'm trying to say that you should avoid having the tasty meal as 'the grand prize,' as the reward you get anytime you accomplish something. Reward yourself with a nice piece of clothing, a video game, or an instrument; go to a movie or take a trip to the amusement park or a museum—anything you enjoy! Just try to avoid getting high on food. The more consistent you are with the behavior you show during your strictest periods, the better you'll feel in the medium to long term, and the more results you'll achieve during your lifetime. The increase in calories will make you happy as shit, so don't worry about having to be strict or boring—you're being consistent and smart about your food.

Just because we're starting the recalibration period in a cautionary manner, doesn't mean you should enjoy life any less than you've planned to. You *should* enjoy tasty meals and drinks during these times, and you should do so without anxiety and having to think too much about it. The key point is that you let such times be exceptions.

If you consistently do what you're supposed to for most of your time, you're allowed to choose your exceptions. One of my best recommendations, which I want to leave you with, is this: save the pleasurable, food-related moments for important social gatherings, where the company itself is more important than the food. If the taste and comfort of food is never your priority, you'll reduce the risk of developing destructive food-related habits.

As you're in the midst of your reset period, a few aspects of your life may start feeling a bit different than they have during the last few months. For one, the increased energy that's fueled by extra calories is likely to affect your mood and general outlook on life. Enjoy it! Just remember that more calories won't sustain an upward happiness curve. The (authentic) experience of being happy and energized right around this time is so pronounced because the contrast to recent months is so strong. More calories and healthy food won't strengthen or lengthen these emotions, so don't try to ride the happiness wave, just enjoy that you experience it, if that makes any sense.

Again, what you've achieved is commendable. Congratulations! Now, celebrate!

A Lesson on Food as Fuel

It all depends on how you've been eating during your reset, but a few days into it is when the most euphoric food-related experiences are turning back to normal. It's one of those things: the hungrier you are, the better the food tastes. When fully satisfied, it takes one hell of a snack to recreate the experience you had on your first bite.

The same goes for the larger perspective, although the contrasts aren't as sharp. Being able to eat whatever you're in the mood for is fantastic for a few days, but soon enough the pleasure diminishes. After a few months with such a routine, the effect tends to reverse into anxiety, not to speak of the physical side-effects.

So, what am I saying? Well, tasty food won't be a friend or a comfort in the long run. Tasty food is something to enjoy at times, not something to strive to eat during all meals, all the time. I've lived with the latter type of mindset, and I've seen what it can lead to, which is why I want to stress this point. Just after a drastic transformation, similar to the one you've been going through, I thought I could eat whatever I wanted, all the time, until I wanted to get back into shape again. I had four fun days, then the euphoria started reversing. It took a long time to get back to sound food routines, and the effort it took wasn't worth the four fun days.

The primary lesson I learned from the experience I had, which I want to pass on, is that food is better likened to fuel for your body and mind than anything else. Here's how I've chosen to see it: your body always needs fuel, and it's always best to eat the most nutritious food in the right quantity for you; therefore, I try to eat like this as consistently as possible. Your mind sometimes needs fuel too, however, and it's not always the most nutritious food your mind craves to settle down. If you, like me, at times want a pizza because you haven't had one in a while, I say go for it. The key is that you stay as consistent with the 'fuel' habits as possible and save the tasty meals for when you allow yourself exceptions.

It's no point wishing you could be eating precisely what you crave all the time. There's no constant food heaven—it's an illusion. The pleasurable effect wears off quickly, and it eventually starts to reverse. Try instead to see food as fuel rather than as a reward for good behavior or a comfort when things are going badly. If you always strive to give your body as much good fuel as possible, in the right amounts, as consistently as possible, you can enjoy whatever you like from time to time.

The New Starting Point

With a full stomach and good progress in recent memory, managing everyday life and doing enough on a daily basis is a piece of cake. As long as you're not actively trying to eat everything in sight, you'll be alright, basically.

It's precisely because of this current lack of resistance that I'll be hyping up the idea of implementing exercise into your life during this reset. We're currently able to add more new ideas and activities, and things will feel similar anyway. This is why *habit* is such a crucial (and interesting) concept. When habit makes itself apparent, things start to feel easy, even too easy.

When we've reduced something that's previously been challenging (controlling and transforming your body) to something more resembling a simple task, there's room to fill out the void that we've created. This is how musicians develop too. When striking a G-chord on the guitar doesn't take forty seconds to achieve—when it instead has become habitual and unrestrained by the development of habit—there's mental capacity and room to focus on producing simultaneous vocals over the guitar chords.

When you no longer struggle with calorie counting, tracking, and target setting, there's room to experiment with many more types of food, various side activities, or simply room to focus on what to do with the extra time that comes from not eating at all times of the day and being able to eat what you should without spending excess time or mental energy on this task.

Being able to develop (the right) habits is the key to controlling your body, as well as many other areas of your life. When a challenge starts feeling like a simple task, you know that you've made progress. Either enjoy the simplicity you've created or fill the void with another beneficial practice that can turn into a habit.

Your Optional but Highly Recommended Task—Exercise

So, with the idea of habits in mind, I'll now introduce the main task that I recommend to anyone who has managed to habitualize the food-related aspects already. One of the best and most practical activities on which you can spend the extra energy you currently have is exercise. Strength and performance tend to develop very well when excess calories and continuity are blended.

If you haven't made exercise a habit and a routine yet, this is simply a great time to start. If you already dabble in it, this is the time to take it to the next level. Do feel free to go back and have a look at previous chapters if you want to refresh your mind about exercise. Adding muscle and strength will not only improve your appearance significantly, but it will do tremendous good to your overall health too. Don't underestimate the benefits of exercise, both now and in the long run.

Here's the thing: muscle is kind of like clay with which you can sculpt and shape your body. Comparatively, the process of transforming, which you now are very familiar with, is a tool that helps reveal what your body actually looks like. Combine the ability to manage your weight and body fat levels with the ability to change the size and proportions of various areas of your body, and you have every single tool you would ever need to achieve your ideal physique! Let both processes take their time and pursue them for the long term. The reward for the patient and consistent is a decade or three of yearly improvements, both health-wise and appearance-wise, so don't underestimate the power of eating with awareness, and exercising consistently.

To sum up, the excess calories should provide a few weeks of great prerequisites for exercise, and this applies to both advanced exercisers and complete beginners. When it's time to start the next transformation block (similar to the one you've just completed), there will be a few solid weeks of exercise behind you, and this matters. Either those few weeks form the start of a new routine of exercise or they make sure the strength and performance baseline is as high as it can be before the next transformation block of time when calories will get increasingly lower.

A Good Gym or a Home Gym

Cardio can be done anywhere in the world, and in most places all through the year. Exercising with weights, however, isn't as easy to do just anywhere. Hence, it's quite important to ensure that gym equipment is readily available, one way or another. We want exercise to become a habit, and it's necessary that practicing this new habit is as unhindered and simple as possible. Not to worry, it's very possible.

There are two types of weight training locations I typically recommend: a good gym or a home gym. The most common way people find weights to lift is by going to the gym. That's currently what I'm doing myself, although this hasn't always been the case. For a period of over eight years I've had memberships in around two dozen different gyms in three countries and visited many more. By now, I've seen both variety and common denominators. What constitutes a 'good setting' is a subjective matter. Some prefer one environment to another, and that's that. However, there are some factors that, objectively speaking, indicate whether a gym is good. Here's what I've found them to be:

- The gym isn't too crowded
- At least 99 percent of the equipment is functioning
- There are enough weights to go around
- The gym is well located and easily accessible

As you can tell, a good gym is a *reliable* gym. You want to be able to do what you need to do (do your *enough*), and you don't want to be hindered by others doing the same, by distance, or time restraints. It's as simple as that. The equipment should be functioning and ready for you whenever you need it; that's all you need.

What other place could always be easily accessible and reliably let you do your thing whenever you need to? The home gym. My own home gym is where I built my foundation for the first eight years of my lifting life. All you need are streets to walk or run on, a solid power rack to place your weights on and to remain safe when lifting, an adjustable bench, and maybe, just maybe, a gym carpet to protect your floor. That's it.

An equipment set like this will cost around $1,000–$2,000, depending on brand and whether you can get your stuff second hand or not, which often works just as well as brand-new equipment. You can ignore appearance, just make sure the barbell isn't bent, and that the other equipment is fully functional and safe. You don't need a lot of space to have a home gym. A good estimate of required space, if you want an Olympic sized barbell, is a width of around 10 feet/3 meters, and a depth of around 7 feet/2 meters. So in essence, you just need to be able to fit a rack and a barbell. And, if you split the sum into three to four years' worth of monthly gym membership payments, the cost is equal.

Healthy, Fit, and Good Looking

By now, you may have experienced what it feels like to go through a transformation, as well as what it feels like being full and satisfied again. With those contrasting states of being in mind, I would like to point out something that's not always clear to everyone (myself included at one time): there's a difference between being healthy, fit, and looking great. Sounds obvious, but what does it mean?

In broad terms, we could put it like this: a healthy body is one wherein the blood, organs, joints, and bones are in a good, healthy condition. Healthy people come in many different shapes and sizes, and it's not always easy to tell who is healthy by sight.

A fit body, to illustrate the point, would be one that could perform physically demanding tasks satisfactorily. Being able to run seven marathons in a week, for example, is an obvious sign of fitness. But all the same, running seven marathons is likely to strain the person's joints, skin, and potentially also nutrient balances, depending on what the runner was able to eat during the week of marathons. Consider this feat of fitness from a health perspective. Think about how this marathon runner might feel after having completed the marathons. Also try to imagine what the person could look like.

Finally, a good-looking body can be fit and healthy, but that's definitively not a requirement. Of course, what 'looks good' is subjective, and what 'being fit' is, is relative. However, try to appreciate the following parable: representing a fashion brand on the catwalk requires a skinny look, year-round. If you're not born skinny, your appearance will most likely require years' worth of meticulous caloric deficits. Certainly, many dedicated people (not only models) have prioritized their look before health and fitness—think of actors, or even bodybuilders. When it's time to go on stage, bodybuilders are at their peak when it comes to appearance, but at the bottom when it comes to health and their personal benchmark for fitness.

I intend the above generalizations to serve as reference material for you. They should help you answer the question of what *you* want to achieve. Regardless of how the above comes across, I don't mean the generalizations to be negative, suggestive, or condemning. People choose their endeavor for many reasons. Bodybuilders often find solace in the severely arduous process they need to go through to present a piece of art—their bodies—on stage. A lot of fit people (especially Olympians, it turns out), sacrifice everything they have to 'conquer the challenge,' whether it be running a marathon in record time, achieving a heavy lift, or climbing a particularly dangerous and challenging mountain. Other people strive to achieve a look to match their lifestyle. If the goal is to make your body a great place for clothes to sit on, who's to say you should be fitter?

The only thing I would like to add here is that a basic level of health is required for everyone. The extremes of bad health are called anorexia, obesity, anxiety, depression, and disability. No one can afford the price of bad health. How much is a million dollars worth if you're fully bedridden or permanently mentally ill? A baseline of health is an absolute necessity, no exceptions. How fit and how jacked/skinny/big you want to be is up to you, as long as you have your health.

Don't Get Injured

Rule number one when it comes to exercising with weights is don't get injured. Even though the concept is easy to understand intellectually, the rule itself is one of the trickier ones to honor in the long run.

One of the two major speed bumps that make adherence to this rule difficult is overcautiousness, which affects those who take the mantra too much to heart and develop an unreasonable fearfulness against pushing boundaries (weightlifting-wise). Struggling with a heavy weight is different from repeating an unbalanced lift, which is likely to cause future injury.

The typical person who is overcautious can be found in the gym doing the same three sets of 55.5 kg. (122 lb.) for ten reps without struggling, for weeks on end. If someone eventually were to compliment this person, saying that the weight has started to look very easy, and ask how much weight is going to be added during the next session, the person in question would likely say something like, "I'm going to make sure I can do this weight properly for one more month, then I'll increase the weight by 2.5 kg. (5.5 lb.)."

Experimenting with heavier weights and lower reps would force, in a positive way, the exemplified person's body and mind to adjust to new challenges. The ability to adapt to a new stimulus is highly desirable. A body that can adapt to increasing resistance becomes both stronger and more resilient, not more prone to injury.

On the other hand, there's the other extreme: overreaching. The overreacher is a person who actually does what the overcautious person fears—they do an exercise improperly for an extended period of time and become more and more prone to injury for each succeeding lifting session.

Constantly bench pressing with a significant tilt to the right may cause injury in the long term; the activity of pushing heavy weight itself won't if the lifter doesn't repeatedly lift while significantly imbalanced.

The Partner

This is often a top-tier tip when it comes to exercising and diet: get yourself a great training partner. I agree with this advice when I think about it. Although 95 percent of my time exercising and dieting has been spent alone, the sporadic months with training partners have always been fun and motivating. Perhaps this is an area where I need to improve a lot.

Anyway, the reason I mention such a great tip this far into the game is because I prioritize that an individual learns to be fully independent when transforming, before learning anything else. Although a good training partner holds you accountable for your actions in a good way, and motivates you just as you motivate them, it's still an external factor at the end of the day. Were your training partner to suddenly leave town, and you weren't fully aware of how to achieve the results you desire independently, you would be back at square one.

Possessing the ability to achieve results creates a sense of certainty and confidence. Without the feeling of confidence and the certainty of the fact that results are achievable, it's so easy—too easy—to give up on the process before achieving anything. While a great training partner, indeed, can provide you with extra confidence and guidance, you still don't want to fully depend on the training partner for those qualities. You want a foundation of confidence and ability intrinsically.

With that said, then, should you or should you not get a training partner? Yes, get a training partner, of course! All you want to be wary of is becoming reliant on them. Your independence and ability are what matters in the end—what gets you your results. If you can have more fun with a training partner, definitely go for it! If your partner were to disappear, stay strong and do your thing until you find another one. Have fun and stay consistent is the point in essence!

Experimentation

The reset is usually a good opportunity to experiment with intermittent fasting. Since you can be certain you won't go hungry for the coming days and weeks, it's often easier mentally to fast for several hours longer than usual.

Let's imagine you've got two or three days behind you where you've eaten until complete satisfaction. On the fourth day, the odds of you waking up hungry are long. So, let's also imagine that you've got a dinner with family or friends planned in the evening of this fourth day. It's likely that this dinner will contain more calories than a normal meal would, and that you'll exceed your target calories of a normal day. However, what if the dinner is the only meal, or the only big meal, you have during that day? Best case scenario, you would be able to get the best of everything; eating whatever and still end up fully satisfied, while not consuming more calories than you would on a normal day. Being able to create extra 'normal' days (calorically speaking) by being experimental like this, you're learning to create more leeway for yourself.

The reset phase, including all of its perks, is intended to function as a mental safety net, as well as a tool to help your body recuperate after a long transformation journey. If you know you'll go to bed fully satisfied, you can endure hunger, even quite extreme hunger. That's why I call the reset a mental safety net, and that's why the reset phase is an appropriate time to experiment. You're able to 'mess up' calorically, for instance, and it still doesn't matter. Utilize your safety net and experiment!

The exemplified experiment is one I tend to recommend to most people that are transforming. However, it's just one experiment out of an infinite number. I urge you to try new things during practical times. The reset is usually an opportune time to experiment with hunger and different types of food. Research questions could be: What fills me up? Is 'eggs only' a good lunch? How does a keto diet compare to a wholefoods, plant-based one?

Another opportunity for experimentation is if an unforeseen injury makes an appearance, regardless of it being during a transformation or a reset phase. This is an invitation to experiment with exercise habits and strengthen less-focused-on body parts.

A Few Words on Meal Timing

Timing is a subject that hasn't been very prevalent in this book, and that's intentional. Whether we're talking about optimal meal timing or when to work out, it usually depends on individual factors, and it's very rarely something you ever need to focus very much on if you're considering yourself to be a quite 'normal' person.

Timing is a factor when aspiring to be a high-level bodybuilder or an elite athlete. If those careers aren't yours to pursue this or next year, you don't need to spend much energy thinking about timing (and you can still reach your dream body, so don't worry about that either).

Regardless of the preceding disclaimer, there *is* something particular to say about time. Finding out your strong and weak periods throughout the day is extremely useful. The thing is that people are simply built differently, from the inside and out. Some are at their most productive at night, while others are more productive during mornings. In addition, people's gas tanks of willpower come in assorted sizes— some have more, some have less. What's similar, however, is that when the gas tank of willpower is empty, *it's empty*. That means you're left to the devices of your autopilot.

If you have solid routines and habits, you'll automatically end up acting by your goals. If you're unfamiliar with the field you must navigate, however, you're likely to miss your target.

Here's an example of what I mean. Exercising with weights has been a part of my life for sixteen years right now. My autopilot is set on the gym, regardless of how I feel. Writing a thesis for school is something I'm not passionate about. Getting to it and working on the thesis (not just thinking about working on it), has required a lot of energy and effort. Whenever there was no energy left in my system—no willpower in the gas tank—I procrastinated with the thesis. The only way to get it done was to prioritize it. Working on the thesis had to be the first activity and priority of the day, so exercising and socializing were secondary. This was the only way to progress.

You may recognize a comparable situation, but with other fields as replacements. Maybe your autopilot is reversed, and you manage schoolwork like it's nothing, while exercise is procrastinated about. Perhaps you love your work, but struggle to leave it in time before the gym closes at night. We all have strengths and weaknesses (or perhaps, we all just have different personalities), but it doesn't have to mean we're eligible or ineligible to reach certain goals. We just need to consider who we are and plan our days accordingly. Whenever energy is high (usually we replenish our energy after a night's sleep), we should start by getting the most energy-demanding task out of the way. For me, it was the thesis. For you, it may be the long walk or the exercise.

Start Preparing Now

Even though you might have a good bit of reset time left, it's about time to start preparing your mind for the coming transformation block (the earlier the better usually holds true here). If you're fully satisfied with where you are appearance-wise, you could start preparing for a performance goal or something else that challenges you. Regardless of your intention, the purpose of this chapter is still the same: prepare your mind in good time, in good times.

As you can tell, 'good' is a useful word that can mean a lot of things (just like our usage of the word 'enough' does too). What's intended with the somewhat weirdly formulated statement above is simply that you start preparing for your upcoming project/engagement/endeavor/process, whatever you want to call it, with sufficient time and when your energy and happiness levels (hopefully) are significantly elevated.

The difference between enough time preparing and of opening a Pandora's box on the first day of a transformation block can be (and often is) similar to the difference between waking up rested at a hotel, where breakfast is made and the cleaning service is on its way, and realizing that it's Monday morning, that you overslept, and you better get your ass to work before you get into trouble.

None of the preceding examples reveal who achieves the best results. Consistency over the long term is king, and it will matter more than one or a few optimal days will. It's very likely, however, that one of the exemplified mornings seemed more attractive than the other, and that's the point. Waking up rested, and having everything taken care of for you, is an easier situation to tackle than the stressful one—simple as that.

If we stick with the hotel analogy, we can highlight another aspect of the point I'm trying to make. Let's say it's a weekend, and that dinner with your partner or your friends preceded the night of sleep and following breakfast at the hotel. In the other scenario, let's say it's a regular workday. Now, everyone's different, but I would still bet that most people would feel more creative and optimistic towards the future in the hotel scenario. The point is this: when you're in a 'hotel' state of mind is when you should start imagining what you want to achieve. As you're already aware, there will be ups and downs during your journey, regardless of what you do.

If you're mentally prepared for the fact that every day will feel different, you're better prepared to embrace the resistance and enjoy the process anyway. So, prepare your mind now, when you have the time and when it's strong. The only caveat is that you must stay realistic with your goals. A target weight or a performance-related target is what I suggest. You should be able to track your goal and achieve it. If your best squat this far has been 100 kg. (220 lb.), it's more reasonable to go for 140 kg. (308 lb.) than for that four-plate squat. Am I losing weight or lifting heavier weights are good indicators that your goal is sound and trackable too. Again, be well prepared, and be realistic with your goals.

Have fun having fun, and good luck with your next goal!

The Reality of Getting Back into a Transformation State of Mind

With the previous idea about planning ahead in good times in mind, it's also appropriate to speak about what it actually feels like to start a consecutive transformation journey. Getting back into a stricter caloric budget can be somewhat tricky at times. It mostly depends on how much your habits have changed during the reset period. If there was little to no ice cream in the transformation period, and ice cream every day during the reset, it may just take a week or two to get used to reducing your ice cream again. Our bodies tend to do that, develop a liking for tasty food, just a bit too easily.

Apparently, we're evolutionarily wired to be a bit gluttonous when we have the chance to eat, especially when it comes to "rarities" like sugar—this would only make sense if we were thousands of generations back in time, though. Nowadays, sugar and opportunities to eat are certainly not rare or infrequent. Unfortunately, we're not going to rid ourselves of the underlying force that makes us say 'fuck it' when we're a little bit hungry, not anytime soon. Generations upon generations of ancestors have survived because they were wired to take every chance to eat.

If we do keep our human inheritance in mind, however, it's certainly possible to override the instinct to eat as soon as we're hungry. Being aware and mindful of how and why we eat is the solution.

Another relieving factor is to not let the hunger become so intense in the first place. That's precisely the purpose of the various tactics we tried during the transformation period. Getting used to eating and not eating during certain hours, and to prioritizing filling food over tasty food, reduces the number of times we end up in a 'fuck it' situation. My point is that just because there's a solution to a problem, we don't need to go look for the problem in the first place.

Whether you've had ice cream every day or not, it doesn't matter. First off, a two-week reset won't be too distracting, and then if you really do have cravings during the first weeks of the transformation period, you're still able override the spurts of hunger with thought and common sense (you won't die, etc.).

Talk to Me

If you've made it this far into the book, I would like to congratulate you (once more). Based on how other people's books, programs, and similar health-improvement instruments have fared, I've learned that it's naive to assume that even a quarter of the people go all the way through. In most cases, it's only a very small minority that actually makes it through.

How come it's like this? I honestly don't know, and my guesses would only be speculation. You, however, have made it here, and that's simply amazing! No one can take the effort away from you, and it is crucial that you appreciate yourself for keeping on pursuing, regardless of whether you fell or stumbled, or will fall or stumble. Please, keep being a person that tries their best, because such people not only help themselves forward, they're the people who influence those who are currently struggling to get back into the game too.

However you managed to make it through, I would love for you to share your story. If you made it here, I'm 100 percent sure you know a few things I don't. Everyone is different, and the best way to achieve results is to learn your own path. Bits and pieces of knowledge come from many different people and finally make out your perspective. That perspective is completely unique and could be tremendously valuable to someone out there who might struggle with weight, appearance, or self-image.

If you've made it to here, you're a person that has figured out a way to get *yourself* forward, towards *your* goal, and I both admire and respect that. You don't have to share your story, but I would very much appreciate it if you did so. You can send it to my email: oskar@managingweightandhealth.com or message me on Instagram: @managingweightandhealth.

In Preparation for Your Next Journey

In another few days' time, or tomorrow, or perhaps even a few weeks from now, it's time to go on another eight-week block. When you say 'go' is up to you. The task is just as simple as it was when we started out. Some days will be tough, especially the first ones, some of the middle ones, and certainly the latter ones. Many days will also be good, probably more than half of them. Better yet, the reward is an even closer resemblance to your target physique. Also, this time around, you may also get much closer to (or even meet) your exercise-related goals. The sense of growth is just wonderful, and it's certainly worth being hungry and struggling a bit for.

This time around, calculating calories should be as simple as it ever could be. Weighing yourself every morning, that's a piece of cake too! The ultimate challenge—which has always been the ultimate challenge since the time of the dinosaurs—is staying consistent with your food intake (and now also exercise). It can't be simpler than that.

The thing is, it's always been this way. Consistent and correct (for you) eating behavior causes specific results. Now you understand this and now you're in possession of the means that help you achieve the type of body you desire. How you use your possessions (in other words, whether you're willing to spend the years it takes to achieve a particular result) is a different question. Different goals take a different amount of time and prerequisites. Some goals take twelve years to achieve, while others can be achieved in six months.

Consistently consuming the right type of food and consistently doing your exercise is certainly not always easy, but it's truly always simple. Inside we know what we should and shouldn't eat, because we understand how the calories affect us physically and mentally.

Spending 250 calories on a Snickers bar eventually just starts to feel ... expensive. And that's precisely the direction in which we want to go.

Food and calories, during our transformation block (and ideally always during any regular day too), are intended to give our bodies the most optimal type of fuel we have the energy, means, or knowledge to acquire, while also satisfying our hunger as much as possible.

You're very aware of what to do. Track your calories and meet your target. Do your exercise. Add cardio gradually. Now, GO!

About the Author

In hindsight, it might look like it makes sense that I wrote this book. I can promise you, though, that I never planned for this or thought it could realistically happen, not until the idea started taking shape 'for real' at about twenty-seven years of age. I've already mentioned that a growing sense of duty made this project feel inevitable. That's the real reason the book exists.

With the benefit of hindsight, however, it might indeed look as though it came into existence by means of intentional planning. I happen to have chosen to study English literature, which is usually a pretty useless degree (especially if you go on to work in sales). Turns out it helped me out a lot while writing this book. I'm also a licensed teacher with a master's degree in education. Understanding, from an academic perspective, how people learn, and why it's an individual journey, was also very helpful of course.

Crucially, however, I've found that real-life experience counts for so much more than theories and academia does, and I've got a fair bit of it. In 2009 I won the Swedish sub-junior nationals in bench press, and seven years later I managed to pass the 200 kg. (440 lb.) mark for the first time. While working towards that milestone, I also started learning about altering my appearance at will. It only took one men's physique competition for me to find out that it's not for me. All the same, the experience still taught me what it feels like, physically and mentally, to be very lean and, crucially, what it 'costs' to become and stay very lean.

At the end of the day, my sixteen years of reflection has led me to this thought: it's about *feeling* like you're strong and beautiful, and it's you who decides what 'enough' is. After having experienced first-hand when a family member reveals they've got cancer, having witnessed how chronic stomach issues can make a man in his best years bedridden, and seeing how depression takes a firmer and firmer hold of someone that's been bullied because of their appearance, I've come to believe that some things are more important than others. Instead of trying to look 100 percent all the time, I would rather spend time with friends and family and look 70 percent for most of the year—you can always transform at will, anyway.

One of the key things I've also realized is that it's pointless trying to convince other people that you're enough if you haven't convinced yourself first. It's perfectly fine to want to adjust one's appearance, but it's essential that there's a legitimate reason for the altering, and that there's a firm understanding of when the ideal body has been achieved. If you never appreciate what you do look like, if you always keep striving for more, you might never get there, and you certainly won't be able to convince yourself that you're enough.

Although this book is about looking and feeling the way you want, I still want to make one thing very clear: as long as you have a baseline of general health, which is the one caveat that prefaces my perspective, you're already good enough just the way you are. Doesn't matter if anyone disagrees.

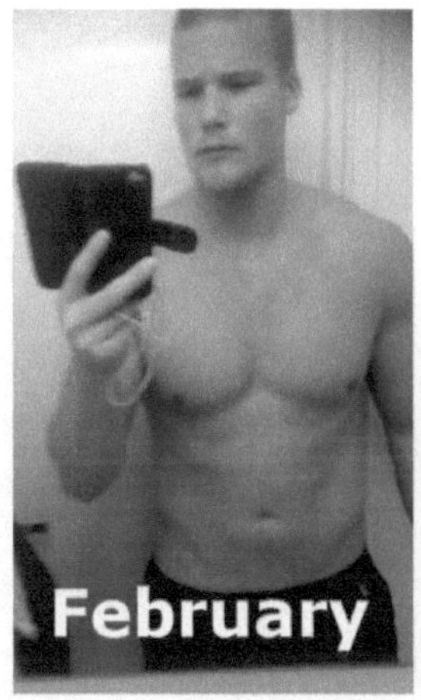

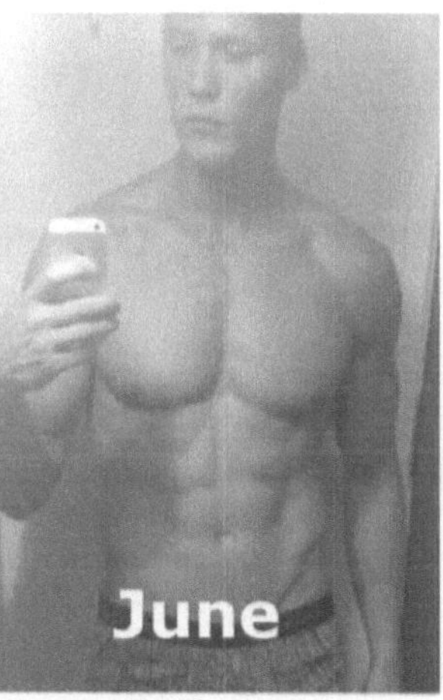

The principles do work, and I use them myself. These are two of my own 'before and after' pictures, just as an example.

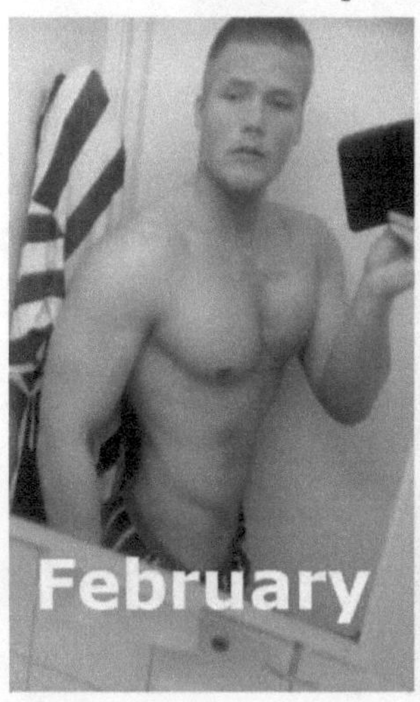

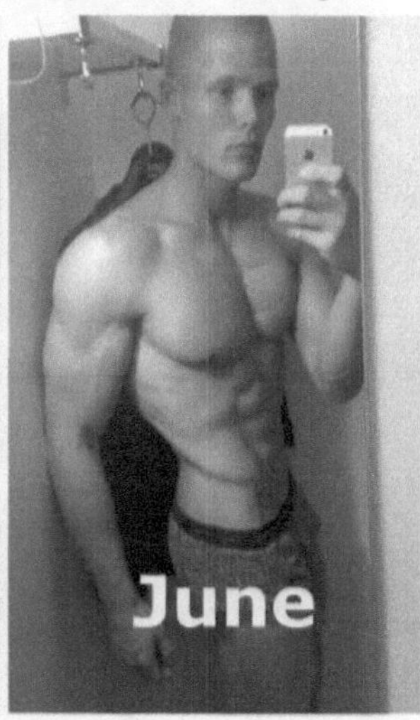

www.ingramcontent.com/pod-product-compliance
Lightning Source LLC
Chambersburg PA
CBHW051441250726
48655CB00001B/182